Occupational Therapist Registered OTR®

Official NBCOT® Study Guide

for the

OTR Certification Examination

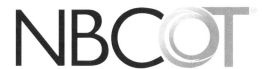

Third Edition

National Board for Certification in Occupational Therapy, Inc.
12 South Summit Avenue, Suite 100
Gaithersburg, MD 20877

www.nbcot.org

NBCOT ... your essential credentialing organization

Mission

Serving the public interest by advancing client care and professional practice through evidence-based certification standards and the validation of knowledge essential for effective practice in occupational therapy.

Vision

Certified occupational therapy professionals providing effective evidence-based services across all areas of practice worldwide.

Accreditation

NBCOT has been awarded organizational accreditation by the American National Standards Institute (ANSI) to the International Standard (ISO 178024) for organizations that offer Personnel Certification programs, NBCOT is also accredited by the National Commission for Certifying Agencies.

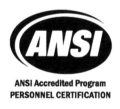

ANSI Accredited Program
PERSONNEL CERTIFICATION

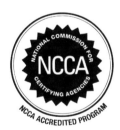

National Board for Certification in Occupational Therapy, Inc.
12 South Summit Avenue, Suite 100 Gaithersburg, MD 20877
http://www.nbcot.org
Printed in the United States of America.

ISBN 978-0-9910328-1-5

▶ Foreword

The National Board for Certification in Occupational Therapy, Inc. NBCOT® is pleased to publish the newest edition of The *Official NBCOT Study Guide*. The occupational therapy content of this guide is aligned to the examination test specifications of the most current OCCUPATIONAL THERAPIST REGISTERED® (OTR) Practice Analysis Study. This study identifies the domains, tasks, and knowledge required for occupational therapy practice.

The purpose of the OTR study guide is to:

* Provide a comprehensive overview of what you can expect during the examination.
* Include practice-focused sample items that mirror ones you may see on the actual examination.
* Outline strategies you can use when preparing for this high stakes examination.

We hope the information contained in this guide supports and augments your overall examination preparation activities. We know the practice of occupational therapy is constantly evolving. NBCOT uses only current information in examination items used for certification purposes. Although the information contained in this guide is current at the time of publication, you must be certain to refer to the most recent editions of references when studying for the NBCOT exam. While the information and practice items contained in this guide can assist your overall study efforts, it does not ensure or guarantee a passing score on the examination.

Best of luck as you pursue your professional career as an OCCUPATIONAL THERAPIST REGISTERED®!

Paul Grace, MS, CAE
President and Chief Executive Officer, NBCOT

▶ Table of Contents

Score Reports
Unfortunate Events

Section 5: OTR Multiple-Choice Sample Items

100 OTR Multiple-Choice Sample Items
Domain 1
Domain 2
Domain 3
Domain 4

Section 6

Multiple-Choice Item Answer Key
Multiple-Choice Rationales and References

Section 7

Multiple-Choice Study Items in Scenario Format

Section 8

Answer Key for Multiple-Choice Study Items in Scenario Format

Appendices

Appendix D: Listing of common:
   Diagnoses/Conditions
   Intervention Applications/Equipment
   Service Devlivery Components
   Roles and Responsibilities

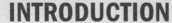

▶ Introduction

Historically, regulation of the health professions in the United States began with a necessity to protect the public from the under-educated and under-trained professional. Over time, licensure, credentialing and certification have continued the tradition of protecting the public but have also increased their scope of activity to continuously improve the quality of practice in the profession.

Certification is a process by which key required competencies for practice are measured, and the professional is endorsed by a board of his/her peers (Barnhart, 1997). Earned certification means an individual has met a specified quality standard that reflects nationally-accepted practice principles and values (McClain, Richardson & Wyatt, 2004). The purpose of awarding the credential – OCCUPATIONAL THERAPIST REGISTERED OTR® - is to identify for the public those persons who have demonstrated the knowledge and the skills necessary to provide occupational therapy services. Certification has become the hallmark credential for professionals in a variety of industries, often serving as a benchmark for hiring and promotion (Microsoft, 2003). For more than 70 years, the OTR "mark" has been recognized by agencies, employers, payers, and consumers as viable symbols of quality educated and currently prepared practitioners.

NBCOT uses a formal process to grant the certification credential to an individual who: 1) meets academic and practice experience requirements; 2) successfully completes a comprehensive examination to assess knowledge and skills for practice; and 3) agrees to adhere to the *NBCOT Candidate/Certificant Code of Conduct*.

Overview and Purpose of the Study Guide

This study guide has eight sections:
* Section 1 contains information about adult learning including critical thinking, learning as an adult, scheduling time for study, and controlling the study environment.
* Section 2 examines strategies for developing successful study habits such as using memory effectively, avoiding procrastination, and utilizing cooperative learning techniques.
* Section 3 considers general test-taking strategies including things to do before, during, and after the test, overcoming test anxiety, and guidelines for answering multiple-choice questions.
* Section 4 refers to exam specifics, including how NBCOT uses the results of practice analysis studies to guide test construction, format of the OTR examination, overview of multiple-choice test items including how to deconstruct exam questions, scenario and clinical simulation item formats, and a sample of a clinical simulation problem. The section also covers information on exam administration.

- Section 5 contains 100 multiple-choice OTR sample items representative of the domains and task areas found in the OTR test blueprint. Although the items included in the study guide practice test are grouped by domain areas to illustrate the type of questions that may be representative of a particular domain, questions on the actual certification examination will not appear grouped by domain, but will be randomized. None of the questions included in this study guide will appear on the OTR certification examination.

- Section 6 contains an answer key, the rationale for the correct response to each sample multiple-choice item, an explanation of why the remaining responses (distractors) in each item are incorrect, and a reference indicating where additional information about the item topic is located.

- Section 7 contains practice items written in multiple-choice scenario format spanning a range of populations and practice settings.

- Section 8 contains an answer key, the rationale for the correct response to each sample multiple-choice item related to the scenario, and a reference indicating where additional information about the scenario item topic is located.

Appendix A includes the 2012 Validated Domain, Task, and Knowledge Statements for the OCCUPATIONAL THERAPIST REGISTERED OTR certification examination. Appendix B includes a reference list of entry-level texts commonly used to reference OTR examination items. Appendix C provides a listing of standard abbreviations and acronyms used on the certification examination along with the associated expansion words. Appendix D includes a listing of common diagnoses/conditions, intervention applications / equipment, service delivery components and settings used on the certification examination.

This study guide is one of a number of official NBCOT study tools designed to assist candidates with their exam preparation. NBCOT does not guarantee enhanced performance on the NBCOT certification examinations for those using these products. However, the official NBCOT study tools are the only OTR and COTA certification examination study tools designed exclusively by NBCOT test development professionals and include sample practice questions written to the same psychometric standards as the actual NBCOT certification examinations.

NBCOT does not administer, approve, endorse, or review preparatory courses relating to the NBCOT certification examinations or study materials produced by other vendors.

SECTION 1:

Adult Learning

Thinking Critically

Learning to think critically is one of the most significant activities of adult life (Brookfield, 1987). Indeed, it can be argued that without critical thinking, the individual views the world through a single, isolated lens, with no awareness of how others view their actions, or respect for the way others behave or make decisions about their world. To think critically is to become open to alternative ways of looking at, and behaving in, the world. As Brookfield (1987) reminds us, it is through critical thinking that we learn to pay attention to the context in which we (and others) think, act, and behave.

Critical thinking should be a core skill for all successful occupational therapy practitioners. It is through critical thinking that the occupational therapy practitioner creates and recreates aspects of the client's life. Critical thinkers are innovators, concerned with the potential for improvement while at the same time, respecting diversity of values, behaviors, and structures that guide the client's world. Critical thinking entails continual questioning of assumptions and an ongoing appreciation of the context in which life occurs. For example, the occupational therapy practitioner will appreciate that a person who has recently become a wheelchair user will experience an array of thoughts and emotions associated with this newly acquired mobility device. The person may feel happy that this device is enabling them to gain access into their community. On the other hand, they may feel embarrassed, or frustrated for others to see that they are having to rely on a mobility device to do the things that they were previously able to do.

All occupational therapy entry-level curricula seek to develop critical thinking skills to prepare their students for successful future practice. However, the skill of critical thinking can also be used as an important strategy for studying and preparing to take high stakes examinations such as the NBCOT OTR certification examination. The following provides a framework of how to apply critical thinking to your studying routines:

1. *Define what it is that you want to learn.* You may be familiar with the anatomical implications of ulnar nerve palsy for example, but want to know more about how this impacts thumb mobility and the challenges posed by this condition for a homemaker caring for a young child. In this sense, you could use critical thinking to help you appreciate the perspective of this homemaker. Define your learning into simple phrases such as:

- How does the impairment affect the homemaker's ability to button the baby's clothes?
- How might this impact ability to carry out grooming tasks?
- Would adaptations be needed to open packets of formula?

2. *Think about what you already know about the subject.* Critical thinking will help you to identify strengths and gaps in your knowledge. Tapping into your previous experiences from fieldwork, labs, case studies, and readings, will give you a foundation upon which to build your learning. It will also help you to identify any prejudices that may be coloring the way you are currently conducting your studying. For example, you may be reluctant to invest much time in considering how you might design a pre-vocational skills program for someone with a substance abuse disorder if you have an underlying prejudice about people who abuse alcohol. Addressing these prejudices will enable you to view situations with an open mind, and aid your studying and ongoing journey towards successful future practice.

3. *Identify resources.* Critical thinking is about recognizing and using all the resources available to you. In this sense, consider resources in the widest possible context, have an open mind. These are a few you may consider, expand on these and design your own list:

- People – professors, fieldwork educators, mentors, peer group, community members
- Materials – textbooks, journal readings, reflective journals, class notes, lab exercises, videos, DVDs or Internet-based search engines
- Environments – fieldwork, community facilities, specialist clinics, adaptive workplaces, inpatient services

4. *Ask questions.* Use your critical thinking skills to enhance your understanding. Do you hold underlying beliefs about this disorder and is this influencing your studying? Does this author have prejudices about the information they are presenting? Is this professor telling you the full story about what it is like living with this disability? Continue to ask questions – why/what/how/if...

5. *Organize the information you have gathered.* Use your critical thinking skills to examine patterns and make connections across your learning. For example, you have reviewed your understanding about ulnar nerve palsy, talked to an occupational therapy practitioner who has provided services to people who have this condition, discussed ways this condition may affect household occupations with your peers, and identified possible short-term and long-term treatment goals from key texts.

6. *Demonstrate your knowledge.* Pulling all this information together, think of ways to demonstrate what you now know. Use lists, flowcharts, and summary statements to highlight key information. Discuss comparisons and similarities of disorders and strategies for overcoming occupational challenges. Write up an assessment report with recommendations for therapy.

Learning as an Adult

Through your occupational therapy education, you will have identified that there are many different ways to learn information. You will also be familiar with evaluating and selecting the most appropriate learning strategy to meet the needs of the clients you are working with. You can use the same strategies to help you identify the best ways for you to learn information in order to help you study for the certification examination.

As an adult learner who has engaged in a comprehensive program of study to prepare for a career in occupational therapy, you will recognize that these are some of the ways you have most likely approached your learning:

- Taken a self-directed approach
- Drawn upon a reservoir of life experiences that serve as a resource for your studying
- Driven by a need to know, do, or find out something new
- Utilized problem-centered, or creative problem-solving strategies to trigger learning experiences
- Been intrinsically motivated to learn as a way to reaching your goal to become an occupational therapy practitioner

It is not unusual however, particularly during transition stages (like preparing to take the certification examination!), for learners to question and re-evaluate their motivation for learning. If you take an adult learning approach to these questions and re-evaluations, it will help you to tap into previous strategies for effective learning, and assist you with renewing your motivation for study.

The following is a list of helpful strategies that reflect adult learning principles:

- *Plan your study.* Take an active role in planning your studying by setting realistic study goals and expected time commitments.
- *Evaluate your progress.* Check off your study goals regularly, demonstrate your knowledge, continually question, and reward yourself for a job well done.
- *Be open to new experiences – people, resources, materials, and environments.* Think outside of the box, who or what could help you learn more about what it is like to have this disability?
- *Recognize the value of past experiences.* Recall experiences from your fieldwork, group discussions, and creative projects. Make connections between these and new learning opportunities.
- *Develop an awareness of what helps you learn best.* Exploit these methods. For example, you may recognize that being able to discuss information in a group helps you to assimilate information. From this, you organize a weekly study group that focuses on preparing to take the certification examination.
- *Don't be afraid to ask for help.* Academic counseling centers, learning centers, writing centers, reading and/or study skills centers, and student service centers, are just a few resources available to students studying in professional academic programs. Adult learning embraces the notion that it is appropriate to ask for guidance to assist with the learning experience.

Scheduling Time for Studying

A common student complaint is that there is not enough time to go around. The time pressures involved in being an adult learner pursuing an occupational therapy education is enormous. Not only does the student typically face tightly scheduled classes, he or she is also expected to carry out several hours of preparation for each hour spent in the classroom, along with studying for tests and writing assignments. This, along with fieldwork and other community-based learning activities, soon add up to a full-time occupation. Many students in an entry-level occupational therapy program find that they have additional commitments related to employment and family/social responsibilities taking up even more of their time each week.

The way a student uses time, or wastes time, is largely a matter of habit patterns. By the time a student is ready to graduate from an occupational therapy program and start preparing to study for the certification examination, these study habits should be well-developed. Inefficient study habits can be changed however, and it is worth reviewing strategies for time scheduling here, reinforcing adult learning principles of taking responsibility for managing time when studying for the certification examination.

Use the following strategies to help schedule your time for studying:

- *Plan enough time for study.* Review the way you have planned your time to prepare for key assignments during your occupational therapy education. Think of occasions when you achieved a particularly successful grade or outcome, assess the factors that contributed to this including the amount of time you dedicated for preparation. In terms of the preparation you covered, knowledge that was being tested, and type of test/assignment given, estimate in hours/days how much preparation you carried out for this test. Now compare this to the certification examination. What are the similarities and differences between the two tests/assignments? Begin to formulate how much time you will need to optimally study for the certification examination. You are your own best estimator, you know how you work, and how much time you will need to prepare and plan for a successful study schedule. Be honest and realistic with your estimation.

- *Study at the same time each day.* To develop effective study habits, or modify inefficient study routines, it is recommended that students schedule certain hours that are used for studying throughout the day, every day. This enables a habitual, systematic study routine to develop and helps to maintain an active approach to learning and preparing for the test.

- *Make use of free time.* There are many opportunities throughout the day when you could take advantage of additional study time. Carry around a small notebook with the lists, summary statements, and flowcharts you have developed from your studying of specific occupational therapy practice. Use time between classes, riding the bus, waiting for appointments, walking on the treadmill to review your notes. Tap into your critical thinking, question your notes, jot down alternative explanations.

- *Schedule relaxation time.* Just as your occupational therapy training has emphasized the need for occupational balance, you should build in relaxation time into your study schedule. It is more efficient to study hard for a definite period of time, and then stop for a few minutes, than attempt to study on indefinitely. Plan for a 10-15 minute break after every 60-90 minutes of focused study. During this break time, ensure that you move away from your study materials, stretch, and use your other senses such as listening to music or drinking a glass of water, to give your mind a rest from the focused studying. Be disciplined however, to return to your study materials after each allocated break period.

- *Review regularly.* On a weekly basis, review the progress you have made towards reaching your study goals. Are you still on schedule? Do you need to build in additional study time? Is there flexibility in your schedule to allow for unforeseen events? This review time should prompt you to acknowledge just how well you are doing and build your confidence in preparing to take the certification examination.

- *Build in time for longer periods of occupational balance.* As well as taking short breaks between periods of focused study, plan for longer periods of "away time" when you can engage in enjoyable activities. Use these scheduled activities as a reward for reaching your study goals and as a way of nurturing your body before returning to your set study schedule.

Controlling the Study Environment

As an adult learner, you not only need to take responsibility for scheduling time for studying, you need to take control of your study environment. Your occupational therapy education has emphasized the importance of considering the environment in which your clients perform their daily occupations. You can apply the same skill to meet your own needs when designing a study environment to enhance your preparations for taking the certification examination. The following is a list of such environmental strategies:

- *Set aside a fixed place for study.* This ensures that over time, this place becomes associated with studying behavior, and it will be easier for you to engage in study activities.

- *Identify factors that increase your ability to focus.* For some people this means making the room as quiet as possible, for others this means putting on some background music. Check if the room is a comfortable temperature, that you have sufficient drinks/snacks close at hand, that your phone is turned off, and that you have all the materials you will need for studying.

- *Be goal-oriented.* Post the goal or goals associated for your planned study session next to your work desk. This will help you to focus and be an effective motivational tool.

- *Get in the study frame of mind.* Use symbols, or rituals, to get you in the studying frame of mind. This might include wearing a particular article of clothing or jewelry, reading a motivational quotation, looking at a favorite picture, or organizing your workspace. Whatever the action, the symbol/ritual will, over time, become associated with studying behavior.

- *Refocus when needed.* If your mind starts to wander, stand up and look away from your study materials. Reconnect with the symbol/ritual you used at the start of your study session. Return refreshed and ready to refocus.

- *Build in regular review periods.* Post times above your desk when you plan to stop and verbalize what it is you have been studying.

- *Put other thoughts aside.* Keep a reminder pad beside you while you study. Use the pad to jot down thoughts if your mind begins to wander onto other activities besides your studying. Once you have written down the thought, return to your studying. This action will help you to refocus, while at the same time, provide a reminder to you later of things you have to do.

SECTION 2:

Study Habits

Section 1 of this guide considered adult learning and encouraged the reader to use adult learning principles, such as critical thinking, as a way to organize and conduct studying for the certification examination. This, along with specific emphasis on taking responsibility for managing time and the study environment, provides a strong foundation on which to develop effective study habits. This next section gives an overview of specific study habits. While it is not intended to be an exhaustive list you are encouraged to use the list as a trigger for examining your current study habits, and as a springboard for considering alternative study methods.

Effective Habits for Studying

(Adapted from Covey SR. (1989). The 7 Habits of Highly Effective People. New York: Simon & Schuster.)

- *Take responsibility for yourself.* Tapping into the principles outlined in the section on adult learning, remind yourself that in order to succeed, you need to make decisions about your priorities. Ask yourself questions such as:

     What interventions do I need to study this week?

     How much time should I spend reviewing my knowledge on spinal cord levels?

     Would it be helpful to coordinate my notes on major mood disorders with the case notes I gathered from my mental health fieldwork?

- *Center yourself around your needs.* Remind yourself, "What is important to me now?" The certification examination can be viewed as the ending of one journey, and the gateway to your next journey That is the end of your academic journey and the start of your professional occupational therapy career. Use these thoughts to motivate as you set up your study schedule.

- *Follow up on priorities.* Keep to your schedule as far as possible. If you have fallen behind, take steps to review your progress, highlight the reasons for falling behind. For example, did you set unrealistic study goals or allow others to interrupt your studying? Try and build in methods to overcome these difficulties in the future such as:

     Reviewing exam preparation goals

     Revising your study schedule to ensure the goals are manageable

     Ensuring the times you set-aside can be undisturbed

     Informing others ahead of time about your undisturbed study time

- *Congratulate yourself regularly.* Remind yourself of the progress you have made to date – the classes, fieldwork, labs, assignments, and tests completed up to this point. Use your study schedule and completed study goals to highlight the progress you are making towards your goal of taking the certification examination.

- *Consider other solutions.* If you are having difficulty understanding readings from textbooks and class notes, think of alternative ways for you to make sense of this material. For example, you might consider talking it through with one of your professors, revisiting a fieldwork site, or joining a peer study group.

Concentrating When Studying

Just as we all have the ability to concentrate, there will be times when it is difficult to remain focused. Our mind may wander from one topic to another, worries about the consequences of not doing well on the test, allowing outside distractions to interfere with study routines, and finding the material difficult or uninteresting can contribute to loss of concentration while trying to study. There are two effective methods for increasing ability to concentrate.

1. *Scheduled Worry Time.* Set aside a specific time each day to think about the things that keep entering your mind and interfere with your studying. When you become aware of a distracting thought, remind yourself that you have a specific time to think about them. Let the thought go, and keep your appointment to worry or think about those distracting issues at the time you have scheduled for these. Let your mind return to focus on your immediate activity of studying.

2. *Be Here Now.* When you notice your thoughts wandering, say to yourself, "Be here now." Gently bring your attention back to where you want it to be – your notes on developmental milestones, for example. If your mind wanders again, repeat the phrase "Be here now." and gently bring your attention back. Continually practice this technique and you should notice that the period of time between your straying thoughts gets a little longer each time. Be patient and keep at it.

Using Memory Effectively

While acronyms (invented combination of letters), acrostics (invented poems or sentences where the first letter of each word is a cue to an idea you need to remember), rhyme-keys, and chaining are recognized techniques for recalling systems or lists of information (and they are described at length in many other generic study guide texts), they are perhaps not the most effective methods for studying and recalling material in preparation for the NBCOT certification examination. Test items on this examination rely on candidates demonstrating their knowledge as it applies to the practice of occupational therapy.

Alternative methods should include using memory of situations and experiences as applied to practice. For example, when studying the ulnar nerve, the student may associate actions of the flexor muscles with specific tasks such as holding a pencil or utensil. Fieldwork experiences may also act as a strong memory aid where students recall working with a particular individual who had a similar disability to the ones presented on the examination.

Using memory in this sense will enable you to apply your knowledge to the practice of occupational therapy.

Thinking Aloud

Through your learning about human development during your occupational therapy education, you are probably familiar with the term "private speech." Private speech is an accepted way for infants and children to think aloud or say what they are thinking as a way of demonstrating knowledge. Children use private speech to practice words, express ideas, form sentences, and as a way to make sense of their external world. Thinking aloud is essential to early learning. As we grow older, thinking aloud or private speech, becomes internalized. However, whenever we encounter unfamiliar or demanding activities in our adult lives, we can use private speech as a way to overcome obstacles and acquire new skills.

The more we engage our brain on multiple levels, the more we are able to make connections and retain what we learn. We can apply these same techniques to our study habits. As well as reading, we can create images, listen, talk with others, and talk with ourselves about the concepts we are learning. Some of us like to talk things through with someone else as a way of increasing our understanding, and others do not need another person around to talk with in this process. Using multiple senses and experiences to process and reinforce our learning is an individualized process, but one that can be very effective in helping to understand and retain knowledge

Avoiding Procrastination

Procrastination can stop you from achieving the study goals you wish to reach. Here are some ways to help overcome procrastination:

Ask yourself, "What is it that I want to do?"

- What is your final objective, the end result?

    I want to review my notes on occupational therapy frames of reference.

- What are the major steps to get there?

    I need to locate my class notes.

    I need to check out the theory book from the library.

    I need to access my fieldwork journal where I wrote a case study using three major frames of reference.

    I need to prepare a grid showing the major frames of reference for my study group.

- What have you done so far?

    I've got the book from the library.

    I've found my fieldwork journal.

    I've bought some large sheets of grid paper and marker pens.

Next ask yourself, "Why do I want to do this?"

- What is your biggest motivation?

    I want to have all the frames of reference clear in my mind.

    I'd like to apply theoretical concepts to practice application.

    I need to feel I am contributing to the study group.

    I want to feel prepared for the certification exam.

- What other positive results will flow from achieving this goal?

    I can talk about my knowledge during recruitment interviews.

    I can use them to aid in selecting appropriate intervention activities in the future.

    I can assist members in my study group to understand the similarities and differences between the theories.

List what stands in your way:

- What is in your power to change?

    If I choose to review a frame of reference that I'm interested in first, it will help me to feel motivated to study the others.

    I don't want to prepare this grid in case I mess it up, but if I draft it on the computer I can build it up gradually.

    There are so many to cover, I'll never get through them all. If I group them together into categories, they will be more manageable for me to study.

- What resources beside yourself do you need?

    I could use some help with drawing up this grid.

    I am going to ask one other member from the study group to work on this with me.

    I am going to look on the NBCOT website to identify study tools available.

- What will happen if I don't progress?

    I won't know this material.

    There will be questions on the examination that I can't answer.

    I will let my study group down.

- Develop your plan:

    Set realistic goals for yourself.

    Define how much time each goal will take to realize.

    Reward your progress.

    Build in time for review.

    Visualize yourself succeeding!

- Admit to mistakes:

> Everyone makes mistakes. It is part of the learning experience.

> Distractions happen. Build extra time into your study schedule, and try to refocus on the task.

> Acknowledge frustration. We all get frustrated at times, especially when things are not going as well as we had planned. Turn that frustration around, and acknowledge that you are doing something about it.

Index Study Systems

Using index study systems is an effective strategy to evaluate how well you know and understand the material you have studied. Follow these steps to build up your own index study system:

- As you read through your study notes, write down potential test questions about the material on one side of an index card.

> Which neurobehavioral deficits are commonly observed in clients who have had a CVA?

> What effect do these deficits have on performance?

> Which interventions are supported by evidence to use with clients who have neurobehavioral deficits secondary to a CVA?

- On the other side of the card, write an explanation to answer your questions. Include references or texts from your academic studies to validate your response. For example:

> Several neurobehavioral deficits and a typical behavior commonly associated with each deficit may include:
> - Apraxia
>   - Motor apraxia: difficulty manipulating an eating utensil
>   - Ideational apraxia: uses a toothbrush to comb hair
> - Body neglect: washes only one side of the face during face-washing
> - Perseveration: repetitively brushes hair on one side of the head
> - Spatial neglect: does not use clothing items positioned to the left side of the body
> - Topographical disorientation: difficulty finding way around a familiar location
> - Visual agnosia: relies on touch to recognize common objects

> (Reference: Pendleton H, Schultz-Krohn W. (2013). *Pedretti's Occupational Therapy Practice Skills for Physical Dysfunction.* (7th ed.). St. Louis, MO: Elsevier Mosby. Pages 866-867.)

- When you have completed writing up a series of index cards about a particular subject, shuffle the cards. Look at the card on top and read the question. Try to answer it in your own words. If you experience difficulty, turn the card over and review the answer you have written.

- Keep going through the deck until you know all the information you have catalogued.

- Carry the cards with you – take advantage of free time to review your knowledge.

- Use the cards to study with your peer group. Test each other, check that others understand your explanations, come up with alternative solutions to the problems posted.

Cooperative and Collaborative Learning

Your occupational therapy education has provided many opportunities for you to experience cooperative and collaborative learning opportunities. This is an interactive learning approach where group members develop and share a common goal, contribute understanding of specific problems, post questions, offer insights and solutions. Many students find it effective to use a similar approach for studying to take the certification examination.

What makes an effective study group?

- Use understanding of group process principles.
- Keep the group to a manageable size (maximum of six).
- Assign a group leader.
- Choose members who will bring specific strengths to the group.
- Empower members to contribute.
- Encourage commitment.
- Share group operating principles and responsibilities such as:
    - Commitment to attend, preparation, and starting meetings on time.
    - Having discussions and disagreements that focus on issues, not personal criticism.
    - Taking responsibility to share tasks and carry them out on time.

Process of setting up a study group:

- Set goals, define how often and with what means you will communicate, evaluate progress, make decisions, and resolve conflict.
- Define resources, especially someone who can provide direction, supervision, counsel, and even arbitrate.
- Schedule review of your progress and communication to discuss what is working, and what is not working.

SECTION 3:

Test-Taking Strategies

The previous section presented an array of strategies to encourage effective study habits. This section examines general test-taking strategies including what to do before, during, and after the test, tips for overcoming test anxiety, and guidelines for answering multiple-choice items.

Before, During, and After the Test

Before the test:

Remind yourself of the progress you have made to date. You have already completed an occupational therapy program. You have taken many academic courses, successfully completed assignments, and passed several major tests. Think back to how much you knew about occupational therapy at the start of your program, compared to how much you know now. View the certification examination as just one step further towards your goal of becoming an occupational therapy practitioner. You have taken many steps up to this point, and this is one of the last steps you will need to take towards your career goal.

Continue to set realistic study goals. Identify your strengths and address any weaknesses in your knowledge. Regularly review your progress, check off your study goals, seek additional help for information you are finding difficult to understand, build in regular breaks, and try to predict how the information you are studying might be presented on the test. Remember that items on the certification examination are mostly practice-based. Although knowing lists and memorizing facts are helpful, you must be able to apply that information to a practice-based situation. Use your study notes, index card systems, study groups, lists, charts, and review papers to learn how to apply this knowledge to practice across a variety of settings and with a variety of conditions.

The night before the test:

* Do not engage in last minute cramming. If you have followed a well-planned study schedule, there is no need for you to do last minute cramming.
* Make sure you know the exact site of the examination center. Estimate how long it will take you to get there and build in extra time for traffic, taking the wrong turn, unforeseen circumstances. Make sure your vehicle has gas, and is in full working order.
* Make sure you have all the documentation you will need to take with you to the test site – refer to the latest copy of the NBCOT Candidate Handbook online at www.nbcot.org.
* Engage in some form of physical activity. This will help to alleviate pretest nerves.
* Decide what clothes you plan to wear – comfort and layered clothing are key considerations.
* Try to get a good night's sleep, and remember to set the alarm clock.

The day of the test:

* Arrive at the test site early.
* Try not to talk to others taking the same test – anxiety can be contagious.
* Take some deep, slow breaths.
* Remind yourself how well you have done up to this point.
* Organize your workspace – familiarize yourself with the computer and ensure you can see the clock on the screen.

- Ask for headphones if you know you will be distracted by others working around you.
- Ask the proctor for a marker board to use during your test time.
- Ensure your seat feels comfortable, and sit in an upright position.
- Advise the test proctor of any problems or concerns you have regarding the test environment prior to beginning the test.

During the test:

- Divide up your test time carefully. There are 2 sections on the examination – section 1 contains 3 clinical simulation test items and section 2 contains 170 multiple-choice test items.
- Take the tutorials before completing each section of the examination. There is one tutorial before each of the two sections. Time for taking the tutorials is NOT deducted from your actual exam time.
- Use the marker board provided to help you organize and clarify your thinking.
- Change your position regularly – stretch, drop your shoulders, open and close your fingers, shift in your chair.
- Read the instructions VERY CAREFULLY before answering the test items.
- When answering clinical simulation problems:
  - Remember you cannot change your mind and deselect an option after you have made an initial selection.
  - Although you can scroll back to a previous section of a single simulation item to refresh your memory on what was contained in those sections, you cannot add or change the actions you selected on those screens.
  - Each clinical simulation problem is presented sequentially and is distinct from the other problems. When you have selected your responses to the first problem, the next problem will begin and you will not be able to access the previous problem(s).
- When answering multiple-choice items:
  - Use the "Mark" button on the computer screen to review items later if time permits.
  - Only change an answer you have initially selected if you are really sure it is an incorrect response. The answer that comes to mind first is often correct.
  - Rely on your knowledge and do not watch for patterns. The test answers are randomized.
- Don't panic if other people in the room finish before you do. You do not need to leave the room until you have used all of the allotted time.
- If you experience a technical problem during the exam, inform the test center proctor.

After the test:

- Resist the urge to talk through test items and potential answers with your peer group. You have completed the exam, and it is too late to change your answers now.

- Resist the urge to open up your study notes, texts, and review guides for the same reason given above.

- Remember, it is against the NBCOT Candidate/Certificant Code of Conduct to discuss test items with other candidates, or to record test information from memory.

- Relax. You have waited for this moment for a long time, you can do no more, reward yourself for completing this stage.

- If you do wish to post an exam challenge, ensure you do this in writing, and within the timelines given in the NBCOT Exam Candidate Handbook.

Overcoming Test Anxiety

It is of course, very natural to experience a level of anxiety prior to sitting for the certification examination. This is a day that you have been working towards for a long period of time, and marks your passage towards achieving your career goal. Your occupational therapy education has provided you with many instances when anxiety has been a natural response—interviewing your first real patient, arriving at your first day of fieldwork, giving a formal presentation in front of a large audience. Remind yourself that a certain amount of anxiety can actually be very beneficial to your performance. It heightens your awareness and enables you to remain alert. Anxiety can become a problem however, if it lasts too long and starts to interfere with your ability to concentrate.

The following are some tips to help you manage your anxiety:

- Prepare, prepare, prepare. This includes following a realistic and well planned study schedule, as well as preparing physically for getting to the test site on time.

- Ensure you have exercised, eaten, and had a good night's sleep.

- Use cue cards to remind you how well you have done.

- View the test as an opportunity to demonstrate how much you know and have achieved.

- Remember, the examination is not designed to trick you.

- Engage in relaxation techniques – visualization, controlled breathing, tensing and relaxing muscles groups.

- Change position, visit the restroom, have a drink of water.

If you notice that at times you have not been able to manage your anxiety levels, and that this has interfered with your ability to perform on exams, seek help from a qualified professional. Your student counseling center, or healthcare provider will be able to recommend help available to you.

Section 4:

Specifics of the NBCOT OTR Examination

Background

Following certification industry standards NBCOT certification examinations are constructed based on the results of practice analysis studies. The ultimate goal of practice analysis studies are to ensure that there is a representative linkage of test content to practice, making certain the credentialing examination contains meaningful indicators of competence, and providing evidence that supports the examination's content validity of current occupational therapy practice. The periodic performance of practice analysis studies assists NBCOT with evaluating the validity of the test specifications that guide content distribution of the credentialing examinations. Because the practice of occupational therapy changes and evolves over time, practice analysis studies are conducted by NBCOT on a regular basis.

NBCOT conducted a practice analysis study of OTR practice in 2012. The results from this study were used to construct examination test blueprints for examination administrations starting in January 2014.

Building upon previous studies, a large-scale survey was used with entry-level OTR practitioners who were asked to evaluate job requirements on criticality and frequency rating scales. The job requirements were classified as the domains, tasks, and knowledge required for current occupational therapy practice.

- Domains broadly define the major performance components of the profession.
- Tasks describe activities that are performed in each domain (i.e. things that practitioners do).
- Knowledge statements describe the information required to perform each task competently.

Table 4.1: Sample of a domain, task, and knowledge statement for the OTR:

Domain: Acquire information regarding factors that influence occupational performance throughout the occupational therapy process.
Task: Analyze evidence obtained from the occupational profile to identify factors that influence a client's occupational performance.
Knowledge: Therapeutic application of theoretical approaches, models of practice, and frames of reference.

The results of the survey were analyzed to identify the most critical and frequently performed tasks by the OTR survey respondents. Weights were then established to determine the relative proportion of test items devoted to each of the four domain areas established for the OTR examination blueprints. Appendix A displays the OTR Validated Domain, Task and Knowledge Statements derived from the results of the 2012 NBCOT practice analysis study. These statements comprise the test blueprint and will guide examination development for the NBCOT OTR certification examinations beginning January 2014.

The percentage of items in each domain area is shown in Table 4.2. These percentages remain constant on each exam form of the OTR certification examination. As mentioned above, there are multiple task and knowledge statements for each of the four overarching domain areas.

*Table 4.2: OTR Blueprint Specifications Based on the 2012 Practice Analysis Study
(Effective for OTR Examinations Administered January 2014 Onward)*

Domain	Domain Description	% of Test Items
01	Acquire information regarding factors that influence occupational performance throughout the occupational therapy process.	17%
02	Formulate conclusions regarding client needs and priorities to develop and monitor an intervention plan throughout the occupational therapy process.	28%
03	Select interventions for managing a client-centered plan throughout the occupational therapy process.	45%
04	Manage and direct occupational therapy services to promote quality in practice.	10%

Exam Construction

NBCOT examinations are "high stakes" examinations. To ensure the defensibility of these examinations, NBCOT applies multiple levels of quality controls during every aspect of the item and examination development process. Additionally, NBCOT contracts with a professional testing agency to ensure adherence to rigorous psychometric standards for the development, delivery, and scoring of the certification examinations.

Each item (question) appearing on the OTR examination has been developed to assess essential knowledge acceptable for entry-level performance by an Occupational Therapist Registered OTR. In addition, the items are designed to differentiate from an individual whose knowledge is acceptable for certification and an individual whose knowledge is not acceptable for certification. All items have been subjected to multiple rigorous reviews. Examination items are carefully reviewed for bias, making sure that the context, setting, language, descriptions, terminology, and content of the items are free of stereotype and equally appropriate for all segments of the candidate population.

The NBCOT exams include a pre-selected number of field-test items on each test form. Although these items are not considered when scoring candidates' exams, performance data is collected and analyzed. This statistical analysis is an important quality control step that NBCOT uses to preserve the reliability of the examinations. Candidates are not able to distinguish between the scored and unscored items. Once a sufficient number of responses are collected on an item, the item statistics are reviewed based on pre-determined metrics. Items meeting these metrics are entered into the bank of items that can be used as scored items on subsequent exams. Item-level statistics falling below these metrics are used to flag items that need additional review and revision before undergoing further levels of field-testing.

In summary, scored items are only included on the examination if they: 1) satisfy the examination blueprint specifications resulting from the practice analysis study, 2) meet development standards described above, or 3) satisfy specific psychometric standards.

Format of the OTR Examination

The OTR examination consists of two distinct sections. One section contains multiple choice test items and the other section contains clinical simulation test (CST) problems. Candidates can take an optional tutorial about the functionality of the test screens at the start of each section of the examination. The tutorials do not count against the overall time candidates are allotted for the examination.

Multiple-Choice Test Items

Each multiple-choice test item starts with a stem or premise. This is usually in the form of a written statement or a question. Stems always relate to tasks and knowledge required for entry-level OTR practice. The following is an example of a stem:

*A client has hemiparesis secondary to having a right CVA one week ago. Initial screening indicates the client is a retired professional pianist, is right hand dominant, and has mild weakness, decreased fine motor coordination, and sensory changes of the affected upper extremity. The client's primary goal is to play the piano at a family reunion in 3 month's time. Which activity would be **MOST BENEFICIAL** to include as part of the initial intervention to support progress toward the client's goal?*

Following the stem, there are four possible response options. From the four options, there is only ONE correct response. The other three options are distractors. Distractors typically represent common fallacies or misconceptions about the item topic. In the sample provided, there is only one choice that represents the **MOST BENEFICIAL** intervention based on the client's goal. You need to solicit the best response based on all the information presented in the stem. The following are the four possible response options posted for the example above:

   A. Turning pages in a music book to select music pieces for a former colleague to perform at the event
   B. Bearing weight through the right arm on the piano stool while using the left hand to play a tune on the piano
   C. Integrating piano keyboard drills into a repetitive upper extremity exercise program
   D. Listening to favorite piano music while completing dominance retraining activities

In considering the response options provided, you should ask, "What is this question really asking?" The question above is testing the skill to choose a client-centered activity that will help the client achieve the goal of playing the piano at a family reunion. You must also recognize the client is right hand dominant, has mild weakness, decreased fine motor coordination, and sensory changes in the non-dominant hand (secondary to having a right CVA). Response option "A" is <u>incorrect</u> because it does not promote progress toward the client's goal. Although option "B" is an activity that may help to increase fine motor control of the affected hand during a preferred activity, weight bearing of the non-involved right upper extremity is not indicated. The client is right hand dominant and has left hemiparesis; therefore, dominance retraining is not indicated. This information makes response option "D" <u>incorrect</u>. Option "C" is <u>correct</u> because it uses the **MOST BENEFICIAL** activity for supporting the client's goal of returning to piano-playing. Although there is never more than one correct answer in a multiple-choice item, you may find it difficult to choose among the four plausible options. If this is the case, re-read the stem and identify the key words such as "**MOST EFFECTIVE**", "**INITIAL**", "**FIRST**", or "**NEXT**". Boldface words in an item stem provide information to help guide your decision-making about the correct answer. The following sample item illustrates this:

An OTR is interviewing an inpatient who had a total hip replacement 2 days ago. When asked about the home set-up and adaptive equipment, the patient states: "I am not interested in this stuff, I just want to get strong enough to walk again." What **INITIAL** action should the OTR take in response to the patient's comment?

A. Use open-ended strategic questioning to better understand the client's perception of the impact of the surgery on performance.
B. Explain in more detail the importance of using adaptive equipment during both the inpatient and outpatient phases of rehabilitation.
C. Reschedule the session at a time when a caregiver is present to provide the OTR with this essential information.
D. Respect the patient's interests to only participate in gait-related activities and discharge the client from occupational therapy services.

The correct response is option "A". This option supports a collaborative approach during intervention planning and should be the **INITIAL** action the OTR takes related to the patient's comment. Options "B" and "C" may be appropriate at a later stage, but they do not address the patient's reasons for not wanting to discuss the home set-up or adaptive equipment. Option "D" is incorrect – Based on the information presented in the stem, discharge from occupational therapy services at this stage is not warranted.

Now let's dive a little deeper and look at a more systematic approach to answering multiple-choice items. This process is called "deconstructing a multiple-choice test question".

DECONSTRUCTING A MULTIPLE-CHOICE TEST QUESTION

As mentioned in the previous section, the key to answering multiple-choice questions, is being able to identify what the question is *really* asking. This is especially important when answering questions that test your critical reasoning skills – where there are several plausible options presented. If you are having difficulty identifying the one *BEST* correct answer and cannot make up your mind between two answer options, try the following steps to help deconstruct the question:

Step 1: Carefully read the question stem.

Step 2: Identify the topic of the question.

Step 3: Start eliminating some of the answers.

Step 4: Revisit Step 1 again.

Step 5: Select the correct response.

Putting it into Practice!

STEP 1 Start by carefully reading the question stem:

> An outpatient client had a peripheral nerve repair of the dominant hand one month ago. During an intervention session, the OTR observes increased swelling of the client's affected hand. The client has not reinjured the hand and has not experienced an increase in pain since the previous session. Which technique would be **MOST EFFECTIVE** for the OTR to do at the start of the intervention session to reduce this swelling?

    A. Perform manual edema mobilization to the client's affected hand.

    B. Apply an elastic support glove for the client to wear during the session.

    C. Elevate the hand above the level of the client's heart.

    D. Complete passive ROM to each digit on the client's affected hand.

STEP 2 Identify the topic of the question

    A. What is the practice setting?

    B. What are we told about the client (e.g., injury, length of time from injury, changes in status)?

    C. Based on the condition, what would we be expecting to see?

    D. What alarm bells are going off based on the information being presented in the stem?

    E. What are your immediate thoughts?

    F. Underline/highlight key information being presented in the stem.

    G. Which words are bolded indicating very important actions the OTR needs to take?

> An outpatient client had a peripheral nerve repair of the dominant hand one month ago. During an intervention session, the OTR observes increased swelling of the client's affected hand. The client has not reinjured the hand and has not experienced an increase in pain since the previous session. Which technique would be **MOST EFFECTIVE** for the OTR to do at the start of the intervention session to reduce this swelling?

Our review here indicates that the client has a peripheral nerve repair one month ago, and is participating in outpatient OT. The OTR notices an increase in swelling of the affected hand. The alarm bell in this case is the length of time since the nerve repair and the increase in swelling compared to the previous session. Our immediate thoughts should be that during this phase of healing, it is not unusual for a client to have swelling – whether due to dependent edema or inadequate lymphatic drainage. But, before proceeding with an intervention option, it is important to determine if the patient reinjured the hand or has an increase in pain. In this case, there does not appear to be additional trauma. Therefore, from the options provided, the OTR should select the edema reduction technique that would be **MOST EFFECTIVE** to use at the start of the session as an adjunct to the activities planned for the remainder of the session (e.g., active and passive ROM exercises).

The question asks which edema reduction technique would be **MOST EFFECTIVE** to use at the start of the session.

STEP 3 Start eliminating some of the answers

Which ones can we strike off right away?

> A. Perform manual edema mobilization to the client's affected hand.
> B. Apply an elastic support glove for the client to wear during the session.
> C. Elevate the hand above the level of the client's heart.
> D. ~~Complete passive ROM to each digit on the client's affected hand.~~

We can immediately strike off option "D". Although passive ROM can improve joint mobility, of the choices presented, this is not the option that should be used **INITIALLY** to effectively reduce the swelling.

Now that option "D" is eliminated, look at the remaining three options to systematically eliminate the other incorrect answer options.

> A. Perform manual edema mobilization to the client's affected hand.
> B. Apply an elastic support glove for the client to wear during the session.
> C. Elevate the hand above the level of the client's heart.
> D. ~~Complete passive ROM to the digits on the client's affected hand.~~

After reading the remaining options, we should also strike off option "B". The swelling has only just appeared. A glove would be indicated if the swelling continued over time and constant pressure was needed to reduce the edema. This is therefore not the action that the OTR should take **INITIALLY**.

That leaves us to choose between options "A" and "C".

> A. Perform manual edema mobilization to the client's affected hand.
> B. ~~Apply an elastic support glove for the client to wear during the session.~~
> C. Elevate the hand above the level of the client's heart.
> D. ~~Complete passive ROM to the digits on the client's affected hand.~~

STEP 4 Let's go back to the question stem and make sure we understand what this question is really asking.

The client is participating in OT after having a peripheral nerve repair one month ago.

The OTR notices an increase in hand swelling.

Which technique would be **MOST EFFECTIVE** for the OTR to do at the start of the intervention session to reduce this swelling?

An outpatient client had a peripheral nerve repair of the dominant hand one month ago. During an intervention session, the OTR observes increased swelling of the client's affected hand. The client has not reinjured the hand and has not experienced an increase in pain since the previous session. Which technique would be **MOST EFFECTIVE** for the OTR to do at the start of the intervention session to reduce this swelling?

> A. Perform manual edema mobilization to the affected hand.
>
> B. Apply an elastic support glove for the client to wear during the session.
>
> C. Elevate the hand above the level of the client's heart.
>
> D. Perform passive ROM to the digits of the affected hand.

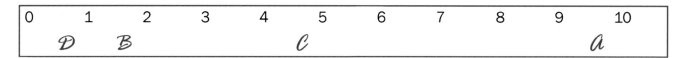

Option "A" is the BEST answer. Based on evidence and the information presented in the item question, this option is the **MOST EFFECTIVE** edema reduction technique to use at the start of the intervention session.

Option "B" should not be done at the start of the session. Elastic support gloves are typically used for reduction of chronic edema. Additionally, the glove may interfere with ROM exercises or other activities the OTR plans to do during the session.

Option "C" might be helpful in reducing the edema. But, of the options listed, evidence indicates this is not the **MOST EFFECTIVE** edema reduction technique.

Option "D" is not the **MOST EFFECTIVE** edema reduction technique of the options listed. While passive ROM is an important part of this client's intervention, this is likely the least correct answer of the options listed.

Using the scale with "0" representing an incorrect decision and "10" representing the BEST option, the "distractors" (response options B, C, D) cluster at the low end of the scale. Response option "A" falls at the high end of the scale based on the evidence and considering all of the information presented in the question.

*References:

Pendleton H, Schultz-Krohn W. (2013). *Pedretti's Occupational Therapy Practice Skills for Physical Dysfunction.* (7th ed.). St. Louis, MO: Elsevier Mosby. Pages 1059-1081.

Cooper C. (2007). *Fundamentals of Hand Therapy: Clinical Reasoning and Treatment Guidelines for* Common Diagnoses of the Upper Extremity. St. Louis, MO: Elsevier Mosby. Pages: 41-42.

Multiple-Choice Scenario Formats

Some of the multiple-choice items on the OTR certification examination are grouped together into scenario formats; whereby there is an introductory passage accompanied by several questions that link back to the same passage. The following is an example of a scenario format:

An outpatient client has a 3-month history of insidious onset elbow pain in the dominant extremity. Evaluation results indicate tenderness on palpation over the origin of the extensor carpi radialis brevis, increased pain on resisted wrist extension, and decreased grip strength on all five settings of the dynamometer. The client reports pain worsens toward the end of working an 8-hour shift as an assembly line worker.

1. Which diagnosis is **TYPICALLY** associated with this client's symptoms?
    A. Radial tunnel syndrome
    B. Carpal tunnel syndrome
    C. Lateral epicondylitis*
    D. De Quervain's tenosynovitis

2. Which of the orthotics listed would be **MOST BENEFICIAL** for this client to use during the initial phase of healing?
    A. Volar wrist splint *
    B. Thumb-opponens splint
    C. Neoprene elbow sleeve
    D. Posterior long-arm splint

3. Which self-administered intervention would be **MOST EFFECTIVE** for reducing the client's pain at the end of the work shift?
    A. Cool water soaks
    B. Paraffin baths
    C. Heating pad
    D. Ice packs*

In answering multiple-choice items in scenario formats, refer back to the introductory passage for key information to assist your decision-making for selecting the correct response. So in the example above, question 2 is testing your knowledge of choosing an appropriate orthotic for this client. The scenario stem provides key facts about the client's presenting symptoms – tenderness over origin of extensor carpi radialis brevis, pain on resisted wrist extension, and decreased grip strength. Based on this information, the correct response is Option "A". Of the orthotics listed, the volar wrist splint would be the most beneficial orthotic device for a client who has symptoms consistent with tennis elbow.

Apply the steps you learned for "deconstructing" a multiple-choice question to come up with evidence-based rationales for each of the response options in all three of the multiple-choice questions in this scenario.

*Note: An asterisk denotes the correct response for each question.

Clinical Simulation Test Problems

Clinical simulation testing (CST) is a format of assessment designed to replicate the types of situations OTR practitioners encounter in their everyday practice. The problems measure a candidate's knowledge and critical reasoning ability sequentially across the continuum of care, for example: screening, formulating treatment needs and priorities; implementing interventions; and assessing outcomes.

Each simulation problem consists of three main parts:

1. *An opening scene*
2. *A series of accompanying sections each with section headers*
3. *A list of decisions/actions*

The decisions/actions list of the CST problem consists of positive, neutral, and negative responses. When responding to CST problems, you should select the optimal therapeutic actions from the list of actions provided. As the action statement is selected, a feedback box will appear. The feedback box provides information related to the action selection. You can use this feedback information as needed to supplement the decisions you make in follow-on sections of the CST problem. Feedback is revealed response-by-response as you make each selection. You will only receive information on the actions you have chosen throughout the course of the problem.

From the list of actions, you score points for positive actions and have points deducted for actions that are negative or hinder the resolution of the presented problem(s). Points are neither awarded nor deducted for selecting a neutral action.

During the course of each CST, you have the ability to scroll back through the simulation problem to view the:

- Opening scene
- Section headers
- Actions selected

This helps you tie decisions to your previous actions. It is very important to remember that once you have checked a decision/action from the section list, you are NOT able to deselect the decision/action. Additionally, once you proceed to the next section of a CST, you will not be able to select more actions to previous screens. CST sections appear in sequential order. You must select your responses to that section screen before proceeding to the next screen. Only one CST problem is presented at a time. The test computer will select the order of each individual CST problem. Although you will be able to scroll back and forth to sections within a single CST, you will not be able to scroll between individual CST problems. Once you have submitted your responses to each section of a single CST, that CST will close and the next one will begin until you have completed all three CST problems.

Key Points to Remember about CST Items

- A CST problem consists of an opening scene with accompanying linked sections and lists of actions.

- When answering CST items, refer to key phrases in the opening scene and section headers to help you decide on the appropriate action options to select.

- Remember, once an action has been selected it cannot be de-selected.

- As you progress through the CST problem, you can tie your decisions to previous sections by scrolling back to review.

- You cannot add actions to previous screens once you have progressed to a new screen.

Example of the CST problem formatting

This section provides some static examples of the formatting of a CST item. NBCOT offers an online CST practice test for candidates who want to experience the dynamic nature of a CST problem.

Note the key components of this sample CST problem:

- *Opening Scene:* This includes general background information about a practice-based situation that sets the scene for the entire CST problem.

- *Section Header:* Information specific to the OT process that is addressed in the section.

- *Action Statements:* A listing of potential actions the OTR will take related to the acquiring information, formulating conclusions regarding client needs, managing the intervention, or promoting quality in practice.

- *Outcome:* The therapeutic outcome specific to each action selected. Note: the outcome section does NOT provide any information related to the candidate's outcome or score on the CST problems.

In this sample CST (Figure 1), the candidate has selected actions "A" and "F" (*note, these are not necessarily positive actions!*). The highlighted areas in the "Outcome" section represent the feedback the candidate received upon making each selection. The remaining areas of the "Outcome" section remain blank since the candidate did not select the "Action" problems associated with those feedback boxes.

Figure 1: Example of the format of a CST Problem section

OPENING SCENE

An OTR contracted to work in a school setting received a referral from a teacher for a 7-year-old student. The teacher is concerned about the student's classroom performance and fine motor skills. A social history indicates the student has an older sibling who has autism and attends the same school. The OTR plans to complete an initial screening to determine the appropriateness of OT services for this student.

Section A

Which action(s) should the OTR to take as part of the screening process? **(Choose all the actions that are appropriate at this time.)**

		Action	Outcome
A.	☑	Ask the teacher to identify the student's favorite storybook.	The teacher reports the student likes to read *"The Cat in the Hat"*
B.	☐	Observe the student participating in classroom activities.	
C.	☐	Complete a review of the student's school health record.	
D.	☐	Confirm the allocation of COTA hours to the school.	
E.	☐	Consult with the school nurse to arrange for an updated visual screening.	
F.	☑	Contact the school district to confirm the number of students currently receiving occupational therapy services at the school.	The school district confirms 14 students are currently receiving services at the school.
G.	☐	Interview the student's parents.	
H.	☐	Observe the student participate in a craft activity.	
I.	☐	Determine the extent of the sibling's developmental delays.	
J.	☐	Review the student's recent written assignments.	
K.	☐	Complete an unstructured observation of the student interacting with family members in the home environment.	
NEXT			

You can now apply the information you just learned about a scenario item to the following sample CST problem (Figure 2). The sample CST problem presented in this study guide closely mimics the format of the computer-delivered CST. For obvious reasons, this sample is not interactive. So consider using the following procedure before commencing with this study guide version of a CST problem:

- Place a note card or piece of paper over the outcome feedback boxes.
- Do not reveal the contents of the outcome feedback unless you select the action as an appropriate action to take.
- Remember, in the actual test you cannot de-select a response!
- Practice this CST problem by only selecting the appropriate actions and reading the feedback associated with those selected actions.

Steps for Using the Sample:

This sample CST contains five sections. The opening scene for each section is the same. Read the opening scene and "Section A" header. Read each action and mark the actions the OTR should take based on the information from the opening scene and the section header. You should use some of the same methods you learned in the de-constructing a multiple-choice problem section of this study guide. Before making your final selections, provide a rationale for why each action item should or should not be selected as an appropriate action. Mark your responses to "Section A" then read the outcome feedback associated with your responses. Considering the information from the "Opening Scene" and "Section A", proceed through each of the remaining four scenes using the same method. The answer key to this sample CST problem is located in Figure 3.

Figure 2: SAMPLE CLINICAL SIMULATION TEST PROBLEM

OPENING SCENE

An older adult is admitted to an acute care inpatient facility following a fall. The fall resulted in a right hip fracture. The patient has a pre-morbid diagnosis of moderate dementia. The patient's caregiver indicates the patient was pre-morbidly dependent with lower body dressing and bathing. A day after undergoing an open reduction internal fixation of the affected hip, the patient is referred for occupational therapy.

Section A

Before meeting with the patient for the initial evaluation, what information from the patient's medical record is important for the OTR to gather? **(Choose all of the information that is appropriate at this time.)**

		Action	Outcome
A.	☐	Review all nursing entries for this patient's hospitalization.	The notes are complete.
B.	☐	Obtain the patient's prior work history.	The notes indicate that the patient worked as a cashier and retired 19 years ago.
C.	☒	Obtain the patient's prior functional level.	The notes indicate that the patient required moderate assistance for most multi-step ADL tasks.
D.	☒	Note the patient's prior social and living history.	The notes indicate that the patient lives locally in a one-story ranch-style home with an adult child who is the primary caregiver.
E.	☒	Note if the patient has a history of falls.	The notes indicate no record of patient falls.
F.	☐	Note if the family has a history of osteoporosis disease.	The notes do not include this information.
G.	☒	Review the patient's weight-bearing status.	The notes indicate that the patient is restricted to partial weight-bearing status on the operated limb.
NEXT			

Section B

Following the review of the patient's medical record, the OTR begins the patient's evaluation. What actions should the OTR include to assess this patient's condition? **(Choose all of those actions that are appropriate at this time.)**

		Action	Outcome
A.	☐	Assess the patient's ability to complete lower extremity dressing adhering to total hip precautions.	The patient cannot follow the hip precautions and the assessment is terminated.
B.	⊠	Educate the patient on transfers from wheelchair to shower seat.	The patient indicates understanding of the procedures.
C.	⊠	Assess the patient's ability to use the nurse call button.	The patient is able to complete this task independently.
D.	⊠	With the head of the bed elevated between 75°and 90°, provide the patient with set-up to complete a grooming task.	The patient requires verbal prompting to initiate and complete the grooming task.
E.	☐	With the patient sitting bedside, provide an ADL checklist for the patient to complete.	After verbal prompting, the patient indicates ability to complete all ADL tasks independently.
NEXT			

Section C

The family's discharge preference for the patient is direct discharge home from the acute care inpatient facility. The patient's primary caregiver will be providing 24-hour caregiver assistance to the patient. In preparation for discharge, the caregiver agrees to participate in the patient's treatment sessions. What ADL interventions should the OTR select for the patient's initial treatment sessions? **(Choose all of those interventions that are appropriate at this time.)**

		Action	Outcome
A.	☐	Demonstrate the completion of transfers from the bed to a bedside commode using verbal and visual cues.	The caregiver demonstrates understanding and agrees to follow the guidelines.
B.	☐	Instruct the caregiver to place socks on client before applying shoes.	The caregiver demonstrates understanding and agrees to follow the guidelines.
C.	☐	Demonstrate the completion of transfers in and out of a vehicle.	The caregiver demonstrates understanding and agrees to follow the guidelines.
D.	☐	Observe the caregiver assisting the patient in the completion of transfers from the bed to a bedside commode.	The caregiver safely assists the patient in the completion of transfers following the guidelines.
▼	*Additional Options on the Next Page.*		

		Action	Outcome
E.	☐	Instruct the patient on the completion of teeth-brushing activities while standing at the sink.	The patient refuses to complete this activity due to pain, but accepts written informational handouts on the activity.
F.	☑	Instruct the patient and the caregiver on minimizing environmental hazards in the home.	The patient and caregiver accept written informational handouts on minimizing hazards.
G.	☐	Instruct the patient on lower extremity dressing in compliance with post-surgical hip precaution guidelines.	The patient accepts written informational handouts on the precautions.
NEXT			

Section D

In readiness for the patient's upcoming discharge, which pieces of durable medical/adaptive equipment should the OTR recommend the caregiver have available at the patient's home? **(Choose all of the equipment that is appropriate at this time.)**

		Action	Outcome
A.	☐	Dressing stick and sock aid	The caregiver would like more instruction about how to use this equipment.
B.	☑	Hand-held shower attachment	The caregiver states the home shower will accommodate this attachment.
C.	☐	Long-handled sponge	The caregiver agrees this will be helpful for the patient during bathing.
D.	☐	Overhead trapeze	The caregiver will contact the durable medical equipment company to inquire about this device.
E.	☐	Quad cane	The caregiver will be talking with Physical Therapy about walking aids.
F.	☑	Three-in-one commode	The caregiver asks for clarification on the best location in the home to place this device.
G.	☑	Transfer tub bench and grab bars	The caregiver has arranged for installation of grab bars.
NEXT			

Section E

On the day of discharge, the patient's primary caregiver mentions managing the patient's dementia is stressful at times. What recommendations should the OTR offer to the caregiver to address the situation? **(Choose all of those recommendations that are appropriate at this time.)**

		Action	Outcome
A.	☐	Advise the caregiver to consider moving the patient to a skilled nursing facility.	The caregiver indicates that moving the patient is not an option.
B.	☑	Contact community respite agencies to determine available service options.	The caregiver asks for help in obtaining this information.
C.	☑	Suggest the caregiver join a caregiver support group.	The caregiver indicates interest in this recommendation.
D.	☐	Recommend the caregiver make an appointment with a mental health professional to talk about these stressors.	The caregiver wants to try other alternatives before scheduling this appointment.
E.	☐	Suggest the caregiver start an Internet-based caregiver support group.	The caregiver does not like to use the Internet.
F.	☑	Develop a consistent schedule for the patient's daily routines.	The caregiver develops a schedule for the OTR to review.
G.	☐	Ask family members to assist in the provision of respite services for the patient.	The caregiver will contact family in the area to see if they can assist.

NEXT

Figure 3: Answer Key and Reference for Clinical Simulation Test Sample Problem

Key	Positive	Negative	Neutral
Section A	C, D, E, G	A, F	B
Section B	B, D	A, E	C
Section C	A, D, F	C, E, G	B
Section D	B, F, G	A, D, E	C
Section E	C, F, G	A, D, E	B

References: Pendleton H, Schultz-Krohn W. (2013). *Pedretti's Occupational Therapy Practice Skills for Physical Dysfunction*. (7th ed.). St. Louis, MO: Elsevier Mosby.

Standard Setting, Equating, and Scoring

All NBCOT certification examinations are criterion referenced. This means in order to pass the examination, the candidate must obtain a score equal to – or higher than – the minimum passing score. The minimum passing score represents an absolute standard and does not depend on the performance of other candidates taking the same examination. The minimum passing score on the OTR certification examination is set by content experts using widely recognized standard setting methodologies.

NBCOT uses a scaled scoring procedure to determine a candidate's final score. The scaled score is not a "number correct" or "percent correct" score. Raw scores are converted to scale scores that represent equivalent levels of achievement regardless of test form. The passing point for the OTR certification examination is set at 450 points with the lowest possible score set at 300 and the highest possible score set at 600 points. Candidates must obtain a scaled score of at least 450 points in order to pass the examination. Additional information about the psychometric principles NBCOT uses for certification examination development and scoring is located in the NBCOT publication titled: *Foundations of the NBCOT Certification Examinations*. This document can be viewed / downloaded from the "Publications" section of the NBCOT website (www.nbcot.org).

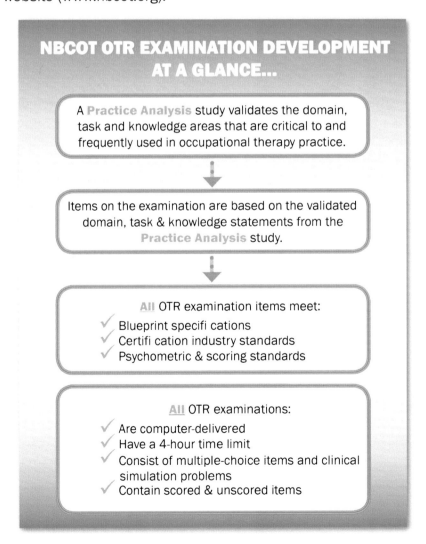

NBCOT OTR EXAMINATION DEVELOPMENT AT A GLANCE...

A **Practice Analysis** study validates the domain, task and knowledge areas that are critical to and frequently used in occupational therapy practice.

Items on the examination are based on the validated domain, task & knowledge statements from the **Practice Analysis** study.

All OTR examination items meet:
- ✓ Blueprint specifi cations
- ✓ Certifi cation industry standards
- ✓ Psychometric & scoring standards

All OTR examinations:
- ✓ Are computer-delivered
- ✓ Have a 4-hour time limit
- ✓ Consist of multiple-choice items and clinical simulation problems
- ✓ Contain scored & unscored items

Examination Preparation Tools

In addition to this study guide, NBCOT offers a variety of resources to assist OTR candidates prepare for the certification examination. Each tool is reflects the validated domain, task and knowledge statements of the current examination blueprint. Additionally, these tools are the *only* OTR certification examination study tools designed exclusively by NBCOT test development professionals. Candidates can be confident these tools provide authentic introduction to the types of questions appearing on the actual certification examinations. For details of the official NBCOT study tools, click on the "Study Tools Central" link on the NBCOT website home page (www.nbcot.org).

The NBCOT official study resources for the OTR candidate include:

- Entry-level Self-assessments
    - General Practice
    - Mental Health
    - Pediatrics
    - Physical Disabilities
- Content Tests
    - Mental Health
    - Pediatrics
    - Physical Disabilities
    - Administration
- Multiple-choice Practice Tests
- Online Clinical Simulation Tutorial
- Online Clinical Simulation Practice Test
- Multiple-choice practice items posted on NBCOT Facebook page

Taking Computer-Based Tests

Test centers are built to standard specifications. NBCOT candidates arriving at the test site must have appropriate documentation in order to be permitted to test. Candidates should check their Authorization to Test (ATT) letter for details of this documentation.

In addition to requiring proper documentation at the test site, NBCOT uses biometric-enabled check-in services at all test sites. This procedure consists of a number of steps to verify your eligibility to test, including taking an electronic record of your ID, photo imaging, and a digital fingertip record. You are required to undergo fingertip analysis any time you leave and re-enter the testing room for validation purposes.

Private modular workstations provide ample workspace, comfortable seating, and lighting (Figure 4). Proctors monitor the testing process through an observation window and from within the testing room. Parabolic mirrors mounted on the walls assist proctors in observing the testing process (Figure 5). All testing sessions are videotaped and audio-monitored. During the testing session, people taking examinations other than the NBCOT examinations may be in the testing room.

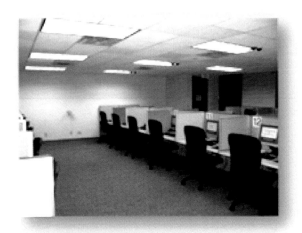 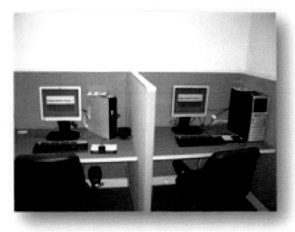

Figure 4: Prometric Testing Center Modular Workstations

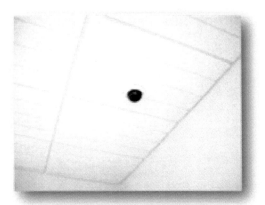

Figure 5: Parabolic surveillance mirrors inside Prometric Testing Centers

As mentioned in a previous section of this guide, the OTR examination consists of two sections: section one contains three clinical simulation problems and section two contains 170 multiple-choice test items. There is a tutorial before EACH section of the examination explaining the process of selecting responses to the examination items. Time spent on the tutorials does NOT count against the time allotted for the examination. Candidates are strongly encouraged to take the tutorials prior to starting each section of the examination. Candidates are allotted four (4) hours to complete the entire examination.

A standard 14-point font is used for the screen text. When answering clinical simulation test items, move the scroll bar on the right of the screen up and down to review all the options listed in the decision/action lists. Once an action has been selected, it cannot be deselected. Once you have progressed to the next screen, you are not able to add actions to previous screens. During the multiple-choice section of the examination, you can use the "Mark" and "Unmark" buttons to flag items, and the "Review" button to return to marked items if time permits. If you run out of time, marked items that have responses will be counted for scoring purposes.

All test situations are subject to some noise and distraction. In a computer-based setting, other test-takers may be taking essay exams, so there may be some keyboarding sounds from test-takers nearby. Proctors are required to walk through the testing area periodically and test center staff may also be providing some brief assistance to other test-takers in the room. If a candidate is concerned that these situations may be distracting, the proctor can provide "noise-cancellation" headsets for the candidate to use while taking the exam.

Candidates may take a break, go to the restroom, or get some water or a snack from a locker. Breaks may be taken at any time, and as often as is reasonable and necessary. The exam time continues to run during any breaks. For more details on test administration, refer to the current copy of the NBCOT Certification Examination Handbook.

Accommodations

In compliance with the Americans with Disabilities Act (ADA), NBCOT makes special testing arrangements for candidates with professionally diagnosed and documented disabilities. Under the ADA, a disability is defined as "a physical or mental impairment that substantially limits one or more major life activities" (e.g., caring for one's self, performing manual tasks, walking, seeing, breathing, learning, working). If you intend to apply for special testing accommodations in order to take the OTR certification examination, you need to provide comprehensive documentation supporting your diagnosis, and the impact of the disability on major life activity. Submit the documentation AFTER you have filed your examination application. A review is then conducted per ADA guidelines. An Authorization to Test (ATT) letter will be sent only after the decision about the special accommodations request is final. Please refer to information about Special Accommodations online at www.nbcot.org.

Score Reports

Passing candidates will receive by mail a congratulatory letter that includes the total scaled score on the examination, an official NBCOT® certificate and wallet card, and the *Credentials Essentials™ Toolkit*.

Failing candidates will receive an official score report that includes the total scaled score, along with performance information for each domain area of the examination. The information on the domain areas is provided for diagnostic purposes only. The score report will include information about how to apply to retake the examination.

NBCOT only provides program directors with a list of the names of candidates who pass the certification examinations. In the event that an education program director requests a certification examination score, the exam candidate MUST grant permission to release his/her score. Candidates may do so by contacting NBCOT to request a *Candidate Score Report Release Form*.

See the NBCOT Certification Examination Handbook at www.nbcot.org for more details about score reporting.

Unfortunate Events

Examination Content Challenges, Administration Complaints, and Appeals

A candidate may submit an examination challenge, administrative complaint or an appeal of the examination score. Details on how to submit a challenge, complaint or appeal are outlined in the NBCOT Examination Candidate Handbook at www.nbcot.org.

Failing the Examination

Unfortunately, not every candidate who takes NBCOT's certification examinations will achieve a successful passing score. While it is obviously very disappointing for any candidate to receive notification indicating failure to meet the passing requirement (a scaled score of 450 points or above on the overall examination), it is essential to address the consequences of this occurrence. A candidate's test score (including a fail score) will only be reported to the candidate, and to a state licensing board, if the candidate requested for their score transfer reports to be sent to a state regulatory board(s). **Without the candidate's written permission, no other persons will be informed of the candidate's failed score.** Not passing the NBCOT certification examination may impact the candidate's plans to begin an occupational therapy job position. If a candidate does not successfully pass the NBCOT certification examination and is negotiating with an employer about a OTR position, the candidate must inform the potential employer about the need to retake the certification exam. Additionally, candidates should contact state regulatory entities for specific information regarding temporary licenses.

Candidates who fail the certification examination will be informed when they are able to submit another exam application. After the exam application has been approved a new Authorization to Test (ATT) letter will be sent to the candidate specifying dates of the candidate's examination eligibility period.

Preparing to Retake the Certification Examination

There may be many reasons for a candidate failing NBCOT's certification examination. Reflecting on potential reasons is an important first step in preparing to re-take the examination. These reasons may include:

- Poor test-taking strategies
- Inadequate study habits
- Lack of preparation
- Test anxiety
- External stresses

After identifying potential reasons, revisit the initial sections in this study guide to help develop a plan of action. Pay particular attention to the sections on Adult Learning, Developing Effective Study Habits, and General Test-Taking Strategies. Use the information from your score report to reassess your knowledge. Review the information about "deconstructing" multiple-choice items. Use this method to supplement further review of the sample multiple-choice items and clinical simulation problems in this study guide. Familiarize yourself with the domain, tasks, and knowledge of the examination blueprint and focus further study on areas of weakness – considering a variety of practice settings and diagnoses.

SECTION 5:

OTR Multiple-Choice Sample Items

OTR Multiple-Choice Sample Items

The 2012 OTR Validated Domain, Task, and Knowledge Statements (see Appendix A) provide the basis for the OTR certification examination item development. The outline for the examination is based upon the four domain areas identified in the blueprint, and the percentage for each domain weight (the approximate percent of items from the domain appearing on each examination) is listed in Table 4.2.

This section consists of 100 OTR multiple-choice sample items across all four domain areas. Examples of domain-specific test items are grouped together under each domain heading for learning purposes in this study guide. However, candidates should take note that the items on the actual certification examination will appear in random order.

The following multiple-choice items are samples related to Domain 1:

> **Acquire information regarding the factors that influence occupational performance throughout the occupational therapy process.**

1. Which dressing task requires the **MOST** challenging integration of performance skills and patterns for a typically developing 3-year-old child?

   A. Finding armholes in a pull-over shirt

   B. Unfastening the zipper of a front-opening jacket

   C. Pulling down a pair of elastic waist pants

   D. Taking off a pair of ankle-high socks

2. An OTR is assessing the reflexes of a 4-month-old infant. The OTR places the infant in sitting and encourages the infant to actively flex the neck forward to look at an object held near the infant's chest. Which of the following responses to this movement indicates the presence of the symmetrical tonic neck reflex?

   A. Flexion of the upper extremities and extension of the lower extremities

   B. Flexion in both the upper and lower extremities

   C. Flexion of the lower extremities and extension of the upper extremities

   D. Extension of both the upper and lower extremities

3. An inpatient had a TBI 2 weeks ago and is functioning at Level III (Localized response) on the Rancho Los Amigos scale. What type of assessment would be **MOST BENEFICIAL** to include as part of the initial evaluation with this patient?

   A. Functional independence screening

   B. Upper extremity manual muscle testing

   C. Standardized visual-perceptual test

   D. Measured level of arousal

4. What critical functional advantage is **TYPICALLY** observed in a client who has a complete C$_6$ spinal cord injury compared to a client who has a complete C$_5$ spinal cord injury?

    A. Improved gross grasp from innervation of the extrinsic flexors

    B. Ability to use triceps strength during transfers

    C. Improved trunk control to bend side to side without falling

    D. Ability to use the radial wrist extensors to supplement grasp ✓

5. A client has a peripheral neuropathy of the dominant hand. A screening indicates thenar muscle atrophy with loss of thumb opposition and palmar abduction, inability to pick up a key or coin from a table top, and decreased grip and pinch strength compared to the non-affected hand. Based on these findings, where on the client's hand would an OTR expect to find sensory disturbances during a Semmes-Weinstein monofilament assessment?

    A. Dorsum of the hand and the dorsal surface of the thumb - C6

    B. Volar surface of the thumb, index, long, and radial half of the ring fingers - radial - median

    C. Entire palm and tips of the index, long, ring, and small fingers - median

    D. Volar and dorsal surfaces of the small finger and radial half of the ring finger - ulnar

6. A client in an outpatient setting has early relapsing-remitting multiple sclerosis. The client lives at home with a spouse and two adolescent children. The client wants to remain independent with homemaking tasks, but finds these daily routines are physically exhausting. What **INITIAL** action should the OTR take to acquire more information related to the client's priorities?

    A. Obtain a standardized measure of the client's functional independence.

    B. Administer standardized assessments of client factors.

    C. Collaborate with the family regarding typical occupational roles.

    D. Complete a client-centered occupational profile.

7. An OTR is a contributing investigator for a unit-wide research project. The focus of the project is to determine if participation in rehabilitation is beneficial to a client's health, well-being, and general quality of life. Which standardized assessment should the OTR use for gathering the **MOST RELIABLE** evidence for this study?

    A. Short Form-36 Health Survey (SF-36)

    B. Kohlman Evaluation of Living Skills (KELS)

    C. Functional Independence Measure (FIM)

    D. Barthel Index of ADL (BI)

8. A young adult client sustained transfemoral amputations to both legs after a recent accident. The OTR is gathering information to identify the client's priorities and personal goals regarding engagement in daily activities. Which standardized assessment tool would be **MOST BENEFICIAL** to use for obtaining this information?

   A. Kohlman Evaluation of Living Skills (KELS)

   B. Functional Independence Measure (FIM)

   C. Role Checklist (RC)

   D. Canadian Occupational Performance Measure (COPM)

9. A client has persistent pitting edema of the hand secondary to mild hemiplegia. Which method would be **MOST RELIABLE** for monitoring the client's edema over time?

   A. Measure the hand circumference at the MCP joint level.

   B. Trace an outline of the hand and fingers placed flat on a tabletop.

   C. Use a volumeter to measure water displacement.

   D. Compare the appearance of joint lines and creases on each hand.

10. A patient in a skilled nursing facility had a CVA one week ago. An initial screening indicates the patient has hemiplegia, ambulates using a quad cane and has good memory. Nursing staff report the patient consistently has difficulty finding the way from the dayroom to the dining room. What type of assessment should be included as part of the initial evaluation to determine the underlying neurobehavioral problem associated with this difficulty?

    A. Functional assessment of topographical orientation and visual perception

    B. Attention and depth perception subtests from a standardized cognitive assessment

    C. Observation of ideomotor and constructional praxis during a BADL task

    D. Cognitive-behavioral assessment of executive function during a familiar ADL task

11. An OTR has completed an initial neuromotor assessment of a 4-year-old child who has moderate athetoid cerebral palsy. Results indicate persistent primitive reflexes and decreased oral motor control interfere with feeding and functional communication. The parents want the child to be able to self-feed, eat family meals and communicate with others. What additional information is **MOST IMPORTANT** for the OTR to collect prior to developing the intervention plan?

    A. Contextual features that support the child's typical participation in occupation

    B. Evaluation reports from other professionals involved with the child's rehabilitation

    C. Early intervention programs available for supporting the child's academic readiness

    D. Medical reports that include the child's past medical history and developmental prognosis

12. An inpatient in a rehabilitation setting sustained a C_7 spinal cord injury 2 months ago. One of the patient's goals is to be able to prepare family meals when discharged home. What **INITIAL** action should the OTR complete to support the patient's success with this goal?

   A. Assess the patient during a standardized meal preparation task.

   B. Observe current physical skills and abilities during a typical kitchen task.

   C. Identify the patient's typical mealtime routines and habits.

   D. Provide the patient with assistive devices to use in the kitchen.

13. An inpatient had a total hip replacement 3 days ago. During an intervention session, neither the patient nor the spouse appear interested in learning about the assistive devices for improving the patient's independence with BADL. What **INITIAL** action should the OTR take based on this observation?

   A. Explore the couple's feelings about using the equipment.

   B. Explain that assistive devices are essential to the patient's recovery.

   C. Advise the patient that the equipment will hasten the healing time.

   D. Document the reactions in the client's record and inform the care coordinator.

14. A client in an outpatient setting has hemiplegia secondary to a CVA. Over the past several weeks, there has been a decline in the client's energy level, ability to concentrate, and interest in intervention activities. When asked about the change, the client replies: "I just can't sleep at night thinking about the burden I am to my family." What **INITIAL** action should the OTR take based on this observed change?

   A. Consult with the client's primary physician.

   B. Advise the client to consult with a psychiatrist. ~only a few wks, not months

   C. Adjust the timeframes for achieving short term goals.

   D. Focus on functional progress to motivate the client.

15. Which of the following symptoms **TYPICALLY** indicates that a client who has been on prolonged bed rest is experiencing orthostatic hypotension?

   A. Diaphoresis when turning over from supine to side-lying position

   B. Lightheadedness upon moving from a supine to seated position

   C. Shortness of breath when sitting up from a supine position

   D. Pounding headache upon moving into a semi-reclined position

16. An inpatient had a myocardial infarction 2 days ago and is beginning phase I cardiac rehabilitation. Which activity is an **ESSENTIAL** component of the initial assessment with this patient?

    A. Identifying stress management techniques the patient typically uses

    B. Monitoring the patient's orthostatic tolerance during movement

    C. Measuring the patient's upper extremity grip and pinch strength

    D. Determining the patient's typical daily energy expenditure

17. An inpatient in a rehabilitation facility has hemiplegia secondary to a CVA. The patient is independent with BADL. The OTR, who uses the ecology of human performance approach, is preparing the client's discharge summary. What information reflects this approach and should be included as part of this report?

    A. Recommendations for home modifications to maximize accessibility and task performance

    B. Exercise protocols for maintaining physical strength and cardiovascular endurance

    C. Current functional status and anticipated occupational performance upon return home

    D. Support groups for promoting the patient's acceptance of the physical impairments

18. An OTR is developing an intervention plan using a bottom-up approach for clients who have hemiplegia and hemi-neglect secondary to having a CVA more than one year ago. Which of the following intervention techniques uses this approach and has evidence supporting its efficacy for reducing the effects of "learned non-use" through cortical reorganization?

    A. Proprioceptive neuromuscular facilitation (PNF)

    B. Neurodevelopmental training (NDT)

    C. Occupational adaptation (OA)

    D. Constraint-induced movement therapy (CIMT)

19. A client in an outpatient setting sustained an acquired brain injury 2 months ago. Evaluation results indicate the client has functional ROM and strength, but continues to require assistance with ADL due to moderate visual and vestibular processing deficits. Which intervention represents an adaptive approach for improving the client's performance in areas of occupation?

    A. Providing the client with an exercise program for improving gaze stabilization

    B. Teaching the client to use proprioceptive cues during functional activities

    C. Incorporating progressively more challenging tasks into a functional activity

    D. Engaging the client in valued activities that promote postural stability and balance

start w/ occupation =
top-down

20. An OTR is using a top-down approach to select interventions for a client who has unilateral neglect secondary to a CVA. Which intervention would be **MOST BENEFICIAL** to include as part of the client's intervention when using this approach?

    A. Determine compensatory options the client can use in the home environment.

    B. Teach drills for practicing head turning to find an object placed near the affected side.

    C. Place commonly used toiletry items to the client's affected side during self-care tasks.

    D. Use tactile-kinesthetic guiding to the client's involved extremity during a dressing task.

21. An OTR is developing a program for clients who are considering bariatric surgery as a weight-loss option. Which type of program represents a comprehensive client-centered approach that would be effective for improving surgical outcomes or potentially eliminating the need for surgery?

    A. Self-actualization education

    B. Stress management classes

    C. Lifestyle modification program

    D. Weekly support groups

22. An inpatient in a rehabilitation facility has a C$_6$ tetraplegia with a rating of "A" on the ASIA impairment scale. The patient has achieved BADL goals and now wants to be as independent as possible with homemaking tasks. Which intervention approach would be effective to use as the **PRIMARY** strategy for promoting progress toward the patient's goal?

    A. Behavioral

    B. Remedial

    C. Biomechanical

    D. Compensatory

23. An OTR completed an initial assessment of a student in the second grade. Results indicate the student has age-appropriate comprehension, visual object gnosia, and visual acuity, but standardized test scores on figure-ground subtests are well below the norm. Which of the following school art class activities would present the **MOST** challenge to this student based on the outcomes of this evaluation?

    A. Painting a free form design on a clay pot using a variety of paint colors

    B. Selecting a round bead from a bag of multi-shaped beads to complete a necklace

    C. Using plastic templates to trace basic geometric shapes on colored paper

    D. Placing tiles of the same color and shape in a straight line when making a trivet

24. A client sustained a closed fracture of the humeral shaft 6 weeks ago. The physician refers the client to OT with a consult that reads: "Begin elbow and shoulder ROM". An initial screening of the affected upper extremity indicates the client has elbow and shoulder stiffness and mild swelling of the hand. The client has full active flexion and full passive extension and flexion of the wrist and digits. Active extension of the wrist and digits is absent. What **INITIAL** action should the OTR take based on these findings?

    A. Focus intervention on resistive activities for strengthening the wrist and finger extensors.

    B. Confirm whether the client has a secondary radial nerve injury.

    C. Fabricate a dynamic splint to compensate for loss of finger extension.

    D. Complete a comprehensive manual muscle test of the affected upper extremity.

25. An OTR is evaluating a client who has an ulnar nerve injury at the wrist level of the right dominant extremity. During which task would this injury be **MOST** evident?

    A. Carrying a briefcase

    B. Turning a key in the car ignition - Froment's sign?

    C. Operating a desktop calculator

    D. Holding coins in the palm of the hand - or ulnar claw - forearm level?

26. An older adult in an inpatient setting has moderate-severe debilitation from prolonged bed rest secondary to general medical-surgical post-operative complications. The patient's primary goal is to be as independent as possible with BADL prior to discharge home. The patient has full passive ROM and Fair minus (3-/5) functional muscle strength of the upper extremities. The patient can ambulate for several feet using a walker and contact guard assistance, but uses a wheelchair in the hospital room and depends on caregivers for wheelchair transport to various areas of the hospital. Based on the patient's current status, which dressing activity would be **MOST** difficult for this patient to complete while seated in the wheelchair?

weakness
endurance

    A. Crossing one leg over the other and putting on loose-fitting slip-on shoes

    B. Putting on a front-opening shirt after reaching for the shirt off a bedside stand

    C. Getting a pair of pants hanging in the closet and putting them on

    D. Washing hands at a sink and drying the hands using a towel placed next to the sink

27. An OTR working in an inpatient rehabilitation facility is scheduled to complete an initial grooming and hygiene assessment with a patient. The patient has mild hemiplegia and neurobehavioral deficits, secondary to a CVA one week ago. Which area of the facility should the assessment take place in order to obtain the **MOST BENEFICIAL** information about the impact of these symptoms on the patient's occupational performance?

    A. Bedside in the patient's hospital room

    B. Fully-accessible common-area bathroom

    C. Bathroom in the patient's hospital room

    D. Simulated environment in the OT clinic

28. A student in the second grade has autism and is scheduled to begin school-based OT. The teacher reports the student has difficulty attending to academic tasks and typically has outbursts when in close proximity to other people. In which environment should the majority of the student's intervention sessions take place?

   A. Self-contained occupational therapy treatment room

   B. Playground in an area apart from other students

   C. Gymnasium when other students are not present

   D. Classroom during routine curriculum-based activities

29. An OTR is developing an intervention plan for an inpatient who has severe post-traumatic stress disorder (PTSD). Symptoms of PTSD started several weeks after the patient was robbed in a convenience store where the patient was working. The patient's goal is to resume work at the store, but extreme fear and distrust interfere with the ability to interact with customers. Which environment is **MOST** conducive for promoting initial progress toward a return-to-work goal with this patient?

   A. One-on-one in the patient's hospital room

   B. During a role-play session in the therapy room

   C. In the hospital gift shop

   D. Discussion group with several other patients

The following multiple-choice items are samples related to Domain 2:

> **Formulate conclusions regarding client needs and priorities to develop and monitor an intervention plan throughout the occupational therapy process.**

30. An OTR has completed an evaluation of a client who has amyotrophic lateral sclerosis. When reviewing the results of upper extremity goniometric measurements, the OTR notes that the client's active ROM is significantly less than passive ROM. What should the OTR conclude is the **PRIMARY** cause for this discrepancy?

   A. Fasiculations   – muscle twitches

   B. Bony ankylosis

   C. Soft-tissue shortening

   D. Muscular weakness

31. An OTR is interpreting scores of a developmental test that was administered to a 3-year-old child. The child scored at the 89th percentile for the child's age and gender group. What can the OTR conclude based on this score?

    A. The child has minor developmental deficits compared to the normative sample group.

    B. Eleven per cent of the children in the sample group scored higher than this child.

    C. This child displays above-average developmental skills compared to similar children.

    D. These scores are sensitive for measuring small changes in the child's overall development.

32. An OTR is evaluating the biceps strength of a client recovering from a musculocutaneous nerve injury. With the client seated upright, the shoulder adducted, the elbow fully extended, and the forearm in supination, the OTR asks the client to fully flex the elbow. The OTR observes the client's forearm consistently moves into midposition on each attempt to flex the elbow; despite prompting the client to maintain the forearm in supination. What conclusion can the OTR make based on this observation?

    A. The brachioradialis muscle is substituting for the weaker prime mover.

    B. The muscle strength of the biceps should be graded as Poor (2/5).

    C. The pronator teres muscle should be blocked on future testing.

    D. The movement should be retested with the client positioned in prone.

33. An inpatient who had a left CVA one week ago is participating in a dressing session. After putting on a sock during lower body dressing, the patient repeatedly attempts to pull the sock up even though it is already in place. What neurobehavioral deficit is **MOST CONSISTENT** with these actions?

    A. Spatial inattention

    B. Somatagnosia

    C. Dressing apraxia

    D. Premotor perseveration

34. An OTR administered a criterion-referenced standardized developmental checklist to a 3 year-old-child who has mild developmental delay. The child did not meet the standard for snipping with scissors. For what purpose would these results be **MOST USEFUL**?

    A. Linking outcomes measures to other typically developing children

    B. Determining developmentally appropriate activities to use in therapy

    C. Identifying functional tasks that would be most difficult for the student

    D. Comparing the child's performance to that of an age-equivalent population

35. An inpatient is preparing for discharge to home after completing 3 months of inpatient rehabilitation. The OTR is reviewing documentation in the patient's contact notes and determines the patient is still working to achieve several short-term goals related to the current treatment plan. What **INITIAL** action should the OTR take based on this finding?

    A. Ensure durable medical equipment delivery and home health visits are scheduled in preparation for the patient's discharge.

    B. Complete a comprehensive re-evaluation to identify current function in relation to the discharge plan.

    C. Discuss options with the interprofessional team for extending inpatient rehabilitation until goals are achieved.

    D. Prepare a discharge summary providing a rationale for the goal shortcomings noted in the contact notes.

36. A client is in the early stages of a slow, progressive upper motor neuron disease. Mild intention tremors and fatigue interfere with completion of typical daily tasks and ability to work a full day as an accountant. Currently, the client ambulates with a cane in the home and uses a wheelchair for community mobility. The client's goal is to remain working as long as possible. Which work accommodation meets the employer's obligation for this client as required by the Americans with Disabilities Act?

    A. Consideration for modifying the client's current work schedule

    B. Employee review to change the essential elements of the job description

    C. Provision of a wheelchair at the job site in case of emergency

    D. Modification of doorways throughout the workplace for maximal accessibility

37. An OTR is planning to give a presentation to a support group for individuals who have recently been diagnosed with a progressive neurological disease. The participants want to learn about the role of occupational therapy in the management of this disease process. What type of information would be **MOST BENEFICIAL** to include to effectively address this topic?

    A. Description of the various types of assessments used as part of the evaluation process

    B. Discussion about occupational therapy for maintaining health and preventing dysfunction

    C. Role-play of an occupational therapy session using a group participant as an example

    D. Outlines of occupational therapy protocols typically used for individuals with this disease

38. An OTR is leading a community-based self-help class for self-referred clients who have rheumatoid arthritis. Through class discussion and observation, the OTR determines that one of the clients in the class would benefit from bilateral hand splints. After discussing this observation with the client and determining the client intends to pay for services using insurance benefits, what action should the OTR take **NEXT** to address the client's needs?

    A. Contact the insurance company to obtain reimbursement authorization for the splints.

    B. Arrange a clinic appointment time to fabricate the splints for the client.

    C. Advise the client to schedule an appointment with the rheumatologist to discuss splinting options.

    D. Complete a comprehensive evaluation to justify the need for the splints to the primary care physician.

39. A patient has flaccid hemiplegia and dysphagia secondary to a CVA one month ago. The patient is participating in an interprofessional rehabilitation program. One of the intervention goals is for the patient to regain independence with self-feeding and become safe when eating. What information about the patient is **MOST IMPORTANT** for the OTR to present to the interprofessional team during each care coordination meeting?

    A. Improvements in upper extremity movement patterns used for self-feeding

    B. Specific evidence-based techniques that are being used during intervention sessions

    C. Positioning, adaptive devices and caregiver assistance needed during mealtimes

    D. Ability to select nutritious foods from the hospital dining menu that are safe to swallow

40. An OTR is completing a functional visual screening of a client who has macular degeneration. The OTR asks the client to pick up a cardboard tube from a tabletop and look through the hole to view a target. The client brings the tube to the right eye. What information should the OTR document based on the client's performance?

    A. The right eye appears to be dominant.

    B. Vision in the right eye is less affected.

    C. Right eye visual acuity is greater than the left.

    D. Focal vision of the right eye is intact.

41. A young adult client has a substance abuse disorder and has been referred to community-based OT. Although the client has maintained sobriety for the past 6 months, evaluation results indicate the client has an unrealistic self-concept, poor social skills and inadequate independent living skills. Which objective would be **MOST BENEFICIAL** to include as part of the initial intervention plan for supporting the client's participation in occupations?

    A. Transition to independent living with a supportive friend

    B. Acquisition of practical skills for basic life management

    C. Engagement in leisure activities with social acquaintances

    D. Education about work stressors that contribute to relapse

42. A client who has chronic low back pain is participating in an interprofessional pain management program. The focus of the program is for the client to learn mechanisms for coping with pain and reducing injury risk during work-related tasks as a manual laborer. The client has been making progress since starting the program 3 weeks ago. What information is **MOST IMPORTANT** for the OTR to report about the client's progress at the next weekly team meeting?

    A. Amount of weight the client is able to lift and carry during sessions

    B. Ability to correctly perform stretching and strengthening exercises

    C. Spontaneous use of self-management strategies during activities

    D. Length of time the client engages in specific work tasks in the clinic

43. A patient who has hemiplegia and cognitive-perceptual deficits has been transferred from an acute care facility to a skilled nursing rehabilitation unit. When should discharge planning for this patient take place?

    A. No sooner than 2 weeks prior to discharge

    B. Throughout the rehabilitation phase of treatment

    C. When the majority of short-term goals have been met

    D. After determining if the patient has potential to return home

44. A patient in an inpatient rehabilitation setting is in the recovery phase of intervention after an acute onset of Guillain-Barré syndrome one month ago. The OTR advises the patient that using assistive devices will improve independence, but the patient refuses to use the devices stating: "My wife is happy to help me whenever I need it." How should the OTR respond to the patient's comment?

    A. Convince the patient to try the devices at least once.

    B. Discuss the patient's comment with family members.

    C. Focus intervention sessions on strengthening and ROM activities.

    D. Identify other strategies for improving occupational performance.

45. An inpatient had a TBI 3 weeks ago and is functioning at Level II on the Rancho Los Amigos scale. Which intervention should be a priority to include in treatment sessions during this phase of the patient's rehabilitation?

    A. Personal hygiene tasks using cueing to minimize outbursts

    B. Simple life skills tasks using compensatory cognitive strategies

    C. Self-feeding program using assistive devices and hand-over-hand cues

    D. Sensory stimulation program using graded and consistent stimuli

46. A young adult client is participating in a community-based OT program after completing inpatient treatment for an acute episode of major depression. Evaluation results indicate the client has difficulty concentrating on simple tasks, has poor personal hygiene, and has limited insight about the impact of the depression on areas of occupation. The client states the primary goal for attending OT is "to get a job". What should be the **INITIAL** focus of sessions with this client?

    A. Assigning the client to a job in a highly supervised sheltered work environment

    B. Finding the client a transitional job involving routine and repetitive work tasks

    C. Determining the client's work habits and current abilities for job readiness

    D. Teaching the client how to locate job opportunities and submit job applications

47. An adolescent was recently admitted to an inpatient psychiatric unit due to symptoms associated with a conduct disorder. Evaluation results indicate the adolescent has a poor self-concept, decreased fine and gross motor coordination, and is socially aggressive. What should be the focus of the **INITIAL** sessions with this adolescent?

    A. Presenting options for pre-vocational exploration and practice

    B. Encouraging participation in self-expression group activities

    C. Providing opportunities for success in a consistent structured environment

    D. Enhancing physical abilities for completing responsibilities at home

48. An OTR has completed an evaluation of a patient who is experiencing complications from pneumonia and was recently admitted to a Medicare-funded skilled nursing facility. The patient was living independently prior to hospitalization and wants to return home. Evaluation results indicate the patient is generally deconditioned and fatigues quickly during activity. The patient ambulates slowly using a walker, and requires frequent verbal and physical cueing for safety when using the walker during ADL. What criteria should the OTR use to prioritize the goals for this patient's intervention plan?

    A. Skilled services the patient currently requires for completion of basic functional tasks.

    B. Amount of assistance that will be available to the patient to maintain progress after discharge.

    C. Patient's desire to improve strength, ROM, and endurance prior to discharge from the facility.

    D. Amount of time the patient will need to maximize strength and endurance prior to returning independent living.

49. An outpatient client has an acute flare-up of stage I rheumatoid arthritis. Initial evaluation results indicate the client's MCP joints bilaterally are red and swollen. The client lacks 10° active extension of the MCP joints on the second through fifth digits bilaterally. The client works as a florist and reports pain as 9 out of 10 on a visual analog scale when completing activities requiring grasp and prehensile patterns. The client will be participating in OT twice weekly. Which therapeutic exercise should be included as part of the intervention plan for the client to complete by the end of the first week of therapy?

   A. Passive motion and stretch of the MCP joints through the full arc of motion

   B. Pinching and gripping a soft sponge in warm water within pain tolerance

   C. Isotonic and isometric exercises of both hands within pain-free ranges of motion

   D. Tendon gliding exercises of the fingers against light resistance therapy putty

50. Evaluation results indicate that an inpatient who recently had a CVA has resultant visual inattention and moderate hemiparesis. The patient wants to regain as much independence as possible with self-care to return home to live with a spouse. Which task should be included as the **INITIAL** short-term goal in the intervention plan when following the sequence of normal development of self-care skills?

   A. Completes toilet transfers and continence management with minimal assistance

   B. Performs bathing and showering activities with caregiver assistance for set-up

   C. Buttons a front-opening shirt and zips a jacket with verbal cueing

   D. Uses assistive devices and compensatory techniques for self-feeding

The following multiple-choice items are samples related to Domain 3:

> **Select interventions for managing a client-centered plan throughout the occupational therapy process.**

51. Which activity represents an effective sensory-based approach for improving tolerance to touch for a 5-year-old child who has mild tactile defensiveness?

   A. Swinging in a prone position in a net swing

   B. Spinning in a seated position on a scooter board

   C. Playing with a feather boa during a dress-up activity

   D. Log-rolling to snuggly wrap the body in a blanket

52. An OTR plans to use a sensorimotor approach to improve the handwriting skills of a 6-year-old student who has a mild learning disability. The student maintains a very tight grip on a pencil when writing, consistently uses a palmar grasp when holding the pencil, and has directional confusion when forming letters. Which activity would be effective to include as part of the **INITIAL** intervention when using this approach?

    A. Painting letters using a wide-barrel brush on paper attached to an upright easel

    B. Rolling out colored modeling dough and making cookie cutter shapes on a tabletop

    C. Using spring-opening blunt-edge scissors to cut out geometric paper shapes

    D. Providing hand-over-hand assistance during writing assignments

53. An 8-year-old child sustained second-degree burns to the first web space of both hands one month ago. Results of a reevaluation indicate the child's web space is contracting; despite wearing pressure garments, using night splints and completing home program activities. What additional action should the OTR take based on these findings?

    A. Advise the caregiver to increase the intensity and frequency of passive ROM exercises.

    B. Begin serial splinting that incorporates a polymer gel sheet over the affected areas.

    C. Provide the caregiver with a list of age-appropriate games that will promote hand use.

    D. Use a paraffin modality during OT sessions to soften the scar prior to functional activity.

54. An OTR is completing a feeding evaluation of a 4-year-old child who has mild hypotonia, immature oral motor control, and oral hypersensitivity. The child sits in a standard dining chair during meals and requires moderate to maximum assistance from a caregiver for feeding. When attempting to swallow food the child hyperextends the neck, elevates both shoulders, and has poor lip closure. What information should the OTR include in the **INITIAL** caregiver instructions based on this observation?

    A. Methods for using cryotherapy to stimulate facial muscles prior to feeding the child

    B. Handling techniques for facilitating full forward neck flexion during feeding

    C. Adaptive positioning techniques for promoting trunk alignment

    D. Neuromuscular facilitation techniques for promoting head and trunk stability

55. A 12-month-old infant has moderate hypotonia resulting in developmental delay and poor oral motor control. Which position is recommended for this infant for promoting oral motor function during feeding?

    A. Slightly reclined with trunk fully supported and the neck and head at midline

    B. Fully upright in sitting with the head and neck resting in slight extension

    C. Seated upright in a standard high chair with a lap tray positioned close to the chest

    D. Semi-reclined in a position of comfort on a soft beanbag chair

56. A school-based OTR is selecting seating alternatives for a student who has moderate hypotonia and has just transitioned to a full-day kindergarten program. The student uses a wheelchair for mobility and does not tolerate an upright sitting position throughout the school day. What type of positioning system would be **MOST BENEFICIAL** for this student?

    A. Lightweight chair with reclining back and reverse wheel configuration

    B. Corner chair with high lateral supports that can be placed on the floor

    C. Dense foam lateral supports and gel cushion for the current wheelchair

    D. Modular wheelchair with tilt-in-space feature in the mobility base

57. A 5-year-old child sustained partial and full thickness burns on the volar surfaces of both wrists and forearms 3 months ago. Although the child wears pressure garments, scarring across the wrist is limiting wrist mobility. Which activity could be graded to **MOST EFFECTIVELY** help with increasing the child's wrist motion?

    A. Tossing a bean bag at a target placed at varying distances from the child

    B. Moving a parachute up and down during parachute games with peers

    C. Bouncing a medium-size therapy ball from one hand to the other

    D. Creeping on hands and knees through a play tunnel maze

58. A young adult client was diagnosed with axonotmesis of the ulnar nerve secondary to a crush injury of the forearm 2 weeks ago. After obtaining baseline assessment information, which technique would be **MOST IMPORTANT** for the OTR to teach to the client as part of the intervention during the initial phase of the client's rehabilitation?

    A. Visual compensation

    B. Hand-dominance retraining

    C. Isometric strengthening

    D. Sensory re-education

59. A client is developing pitting edema of the hand secondary to flaccid hemiplegia. What should the OTR teach the client and caregiver as part of the **INITIAL** intervention for managing this client's edema?

    A. Methods for using elasticized compression wraps for the digits and hand

    B. Importance of proper upper extremity positioning and elevation

    C. Procedures for providing retrograde massage of the upper extremity

    D. Techniques for completing passive ROM exercises of the digits

60. A client with stage 2 Parkinson's disease is preparing to move from sitting on a tub transfer bench in the bathtub to standing up at a walker placed outside the bathtub. Which method would be effective for the client to use at the start of the transfer?

    A. Rocking rhythmically back and forth on the bench a few times

    B. Using a towel to quickly rub the larger muscles of the thighs

    C. Bearing weight through both arms by pressing down on the bench

    D. Pulling forward on the grab bar mounted to the bathroom wall

61. Which of the following joint protection techniques should a client with rheumatoid arthritis use when completing kitchen tasks?

    A. Grasp cookware with the fingertips.

    B. Transport items using a wheeled cart.

    C. Stir foods with weighted long-handled utensils.

    D. Twist a jar lid open with the least affected hand.

62. An inpatient with relapsing-remitting multiple sclerosis has been making steady progress during morning BADL. For the past 3 mornings, the patient reportedly completed the morning self-care routine independently. During a reevaluation of BADL, the patient becomes physically exhausted while dressing after taking a shower and asks to return to bed. In addition to talking with the patient about energy conservation, what action should the OTR take based on the patient's physical response?

    A. Ask the patient to identify the BADL tasks that typically take the most time to complete.

    B. Talk with the patient about pacing self-care tasks throughout the day.

    C. Teach the patient to monitor symptoms while incorporating appropriate rest-activity ratios into self-care tasks.

    D. Advise the patient to complete self-care while seated upright in bed in order to reduce energy expenditure.

63. An inpatient has a TBI and is functioning at Level V (Confused-inappropriate) *non-agitated* on the Rancho Los Amigos scale. Which approach would be **MOST EFFECTIVE** for facilitating the patient's success with grooming tasks based on the patient's current cognitive level?

    A. Provide repeated verbal instructions until the patient completes the task.

    B. Use forward chaining techniques if the patient is distracted from the task.

    C. Demonstrate a portion of the activity then ask the patient to return demonstration.

    D. Give one-step instructions and hand-over-hand cueing throughout the task.

64. An inpatient who has COPD is participating in a dressing session while seated at bedside. While putting on a pair of pants, the patient begins to have dyspnea. Pulse oximetry indicates the patient's oxygen saturation level is 93%. After stopping the activity, what should the OTR have the patient do **NEXT**?

    A. Take several short shallow breaths through the mouth.

    B. Breathe in deeply through the nose and slowly exhale through pursed lips.

    C. Inhale through pursed lips and quickly exhale through the nose.

    D. Breathe through a nasal cannula using supplemental oxygen.

65. A client had an open reduction external fixation of a distal radius fracture several days ago. Evaluation results indicate moderate swelling of the hand, decreased active ROM of the digits, and protective posturing of the involved arm close to the chest at all times. Which intervention would be **MOST BENEFICIAL** to include in sessions during this initial phase of the client's recovery?

    A. Education about proper positioning in a standard pouch sling to minimize swelling

    B. Exercises to promote capsular gliding and ROM of the shoulder of the affected arm

    C. Static splinting to prevent MCP joint collateral ligament tightness

    D. Use of a dry whirlpool modality to manage edema of the affected hand

66. A client sustained a distal radius fracture of the dominant upper extremity 6 weeks ago. A short arm cast was applied on the day of injury and was removed one day ago. The client holds the affected arm close to the chest in a protected position due to pain, which the client rates as 6 out of 10 using a visual analog scale. The hand and forearm are moderately edematous. The client is able to flex the fingers to within one inch (2.54 cm) from each fingertip to the distal palmar crease. The client refused to move the wrist due to pain. Which intervention should be a priority to include as part of the treatment plan during the **INITIAL** phase of the client's rehabilitation?

    A. Fabrication of a dynamic finger flexion splint

    B. Passive ROM exercises for the wrist and fingers

    C. Manual edema mobilization of the affected extremity

    D. Gentle stress loading exercises as tolerated

67. An inpatient is recovering from partial and full thickness burns on the dominant upper extremity and has recently developed heterotopic ossification (HO) at the elbow. Prior to the onset of HO symptoms, the patient was independent with self-feeding. Now the patient uses only the non-dominant hand for holding utensils. Which assistive device would be **MOST BENEFICIAL** for improving the patient's functional abilities when eating?

    A. Universal cuff with elongated utensil

    B. Swivel spoon and elongated utensils

    C. Rocker knife with a built-up handle

    D. Mechanical feeder with supinator attachment

68. A client with a non-operable cerebellum tumor is participating in OT to increase independence with self-feeding. Which assistive devices should the client use to promote progress toward this goal?

    A. Suction plate and cup holder

    B. Side-cutting fork and rocker knife

    C. Plastic cup and lightweight utensils

    D. Universal cuff with mobile arm support

69. Which method would be **MOST EFFECTIVE** to use when grading an activity to improve muscular endurance?

    A. Maintaining the same resistance and increasing the number of repetitions

    B. Shortening the interval of time to complete a controlled set of isotonic exercises

    C. Increasing resistance to 75% of maximal strength and maintaining repetitions

    D. Decreasing repetitions and increasing resistance for short intervals of time

70. A client who had a CVA one month ago now has moderate-severe flexor spasticity and scapular immobility of the involved upper extremity. Which technique is **CONTRAINDICATED** to use for minimizing the impact of the spasticity on passive mobility for dressing and hygiene?

    A. Self-ROM exercises in supine several times per day

    B. Reciprocal pulley exercises using wall mounted pulleys

    C. Upper extremity weight-bearing during functional tasks

    D. Long-arm air splinting prior to completing a self-care task

71. An OTR is fabricating a static splint for a client who has a partial thickness burn to the dorsum of the hand. The primary purpose of the splint is to maintain the length of the MCP joint collateral ligaments. How should the MCP joints, IP joints and wrist be positioned in the splint to achieve this goal?

	MCP Joint Position	IP Joint Position	Wrist Position
A.	20° – 30° Flexion	20° – 25° Flexion	25° – 30° Extension
B.	35° – 45° Flexion	30° – 40° Flexion	Neutral
C.	0° Extension	45° – 60° Flexion	Neutral
D.	60° – 70° Flexion	0° – 5° Flexion	25° – 30° Extension

72. An OTR is fabricating a splint for a client who has a claw-hand deformity secondary to an ulnar nerve injury several months ago. Which type of splint is indicated for this client?

    A. Dorsal-based MCP joint blocking splint with a dynamic component to pull the fourth and fifth digit IP joints into extension

    B. Low-profile dynamic splint that blocks hyperextension of the second through fifth digits and has an IP joint extension outrigger

    C. Volar-based forearm and hand static splint that blocks MCP joint hyperextension while allowing IP joint motion

    D. Hand-based splint that positions the fourth and fifth digits in 30°-40° of MCP joint flexion while allowing IP joint motion

73. An inpatient in a rehabilitation facility is preparing for discharge to home. The patient has hemiplegia, uses a wheelchair for mobility and completes self-care independently with assistive devices. The patient's home bathroom has a standard bathtub and a separate walk-in shower with a safety glass door and a 6-inch (15.24 cm) high doorsill. Both the shower and the tub have safety grab bars. Which piece of durable medical equipment would be **MOST BENEFICIAL** for this patient to use at home?

    A. Padded transfer bench with swivel seat for the bathtub

    B. Shower chair that can be used in the shower or bathtub

    C. Plastic bath chair with armrests and accessory caddy

    D. Transfer board and plastic shower stool with a contoured seat

74. A mobile arm support is **CONTRAINDICATED** to recommend for clients who have which of the following diagnoses?

    A. Incomplete C_4 spinal cord injury

    B. Guillain-Barré syndrome

    C. Huntington's disease

    D. Amyotrophic lateral sclerosis

75. A client with fibromyalgia reports hand pain and stiffness make it difficult to grasp a standard knife and fork during meals. Which assistive device would be **MOST BENEFICIAL** for improving the client's functional abilities when eating?

    A. Utensils with built-up handles

    B. Rocker knife and plate with raised sides

    C. Universal cuff with wrist support

    D. Lightweight utensils with non-slip grips

76. An OTR is teaching stand-pivot transfers to a client who has Stage 2 Parkinson's disease and uses a wheelchair for mobility. After instructing the client to properly position the chair in relation to the transfer surface, and asking the client to lock the wheelchair brakes, what should the OTR ask the client to do **NEXT**?

    A. Scoot the hips forward to the edge of the wheelchair.

    B. Come to standing by pushing up on the wheelchair arm rests.

    C. Rock forward while reaching toward the transfer surface.

    D. Placing the feet in this position presents a fall risk to the patient.

77. An inpatient had a total hip replacement, posterolateral approach 2 weeks ago. The OTR is discussing home set-up and seating options with the patient as part of the discharge instructions. What type of seat should the OTR recommend the patient sit on when watching television at home?

    A. Firm raised armchair with a wedge pillow roll between the cushion and back of the chair

    B. Cushioned, armless dining chair elevated on one-inch (2.54 cm) high blocks

    C. Sofa with enough length to allow the patient to elevate both legs on the seat cushions

    D. Upholstered reclining chair with extra pillows to elevate the affected leg

78. Which of the following environmental adaptations will improve safety during meal preparation for a client who has low vision?

    A. Installing a microwave that has preprogrammed cooking options

    B. Placing tactile markings on the operating features of appliances

    C. Arranging items on the pantry and cabinet shelves in alphabetical order

    D. Using large-sized bowls and pots for mixing and stove-top cooking

79. A client has relapsing-remitting multiple sclerosis and recently transitioned from assisted ambulation to using a standard wheelchair for mobility. A recent onset of fatigue, upper extremity weakness, and back and neck discomfort is beginning to interfere with job performance. The client is employed as a magazine editor, and spends much of the day sitting in the wheelchair while working at the computer monitor positioned at eye level. The client wants to continue sitting in a wheelchair to avoid having to complete transfers when moving from the desk to other parts of the work area. Which modification would be **MOST BENEFICIAL** for this client?

    A. Power scooter with padded seat and electric tilt-in-space control

    B. Voice-controlled computer system and telephone headset

    C. Solid seat insert, lumbar support and bilateral forearm supports

    D. Deltoid aid and a split design computer keyboard

80. A client who is legally blind reports having difficulty locating grooming items in the bathroom every morning, resulting in being late for work. Which recommendation should the OTR suggest for improving the client's occupational performance?

    A. Complete the majority of bathing and grooming tasks the night before.

    B. Wake-up at least one hour earlier so that grooming will not be rushed.

    C. Organize items in the bathroom so that there is a specific place for each item.

    D. Discuss with the employer options for implementing a later start time at work.

81. An inpatient had a TBI one month ago and is functioning at Level VII (Automatic-appropriate) on the Rancho Los Amigos scale. Currently, the patient is able to follow two-step instructions and attends to a familiar task for up to 15 minutes at a time. The patient wants to return home to resume homemaking roles. One of the patient's short-term goals is to independently bake cookies for a family member's upcoming birthday. How should the activity be graded to support the patient's successful participation in this task?

    A. Have the patient prepare cookies using slice and bake packaged cookie dough.

    B. Provide the patient with a recipe of ingredients for mixing and baking cookies.

    C. Have the patient prepare cookies using a boxed cookie mix with pre-measured ingredients.

    D. Mix the ingredients together and have the patient drop the cookies onto the cookie sheet.

82. An inpatient sustained a complete T_5 spinal cord injury one month ago and has been in the intensive care unit on extended bed-rest. The OTR recently initiated a program of graded bed mobility in preparation for beginning transfer training. The patient is now able to sit in bed with the head of the bed elevated to 45° for one-hour intervals without experiencing any dizziness. Which position is safest for the patient to be placed in **NEXT**?

    A. Upright in a standard wheelchair with close monitoring

    B. Upright on a tilt-table at 90° while wearing an abdominal binder and elastic stockings

    C. Seated in a semi-reclining wheelchair with legs elevated

    D. Seated on the edge of the bed with both legs unsupported and knees flexed to 90°

83. An inpatient has been participating in rehabilitation since having bilateral transfemoral amputations 2 months ago. The patient has good balance and Fair plus (3+/5) upper extremity strength, is independent with bed mobility and self-care using adaptive equipment, and requires stand-by assistance during wheelchair transfers and with wheelchair management. The patient is preparing for discharge to live at home with the spouse and an adult son. Modifications have been made to the main entrance of the home and the bathroom. The OTR plans to provide family education for promoting the patient's safe transition to the home environment. What information would be **MOST BENEFICIAL** to include as part of this process?

    A. Methods for improving the patient's independence with transfers

    B. Techniques the patient uses to transfer to a variety of surfaces

    C. Energy conservation techniques for the patient to use during ADL

    D. Wrapping techniques for shaping and protecting the residual limb

84. An OTR is providing a home program to a client who has stage 1 complex regional pain syndrome. What information should be included in the home program to **MOST EFFECTIVELY** help the client with symptom management?

    A. Pictures illustrating passive ROM exercises for each joint of the affected hand

    B. Recommendations for one-handed activities to protect the affected hand during ADL

    C. Techniques for elevating the hand and completing active ROM exercises

    D. Instructions for incorporating energy conservation into daily tasks

85. A client sustained a severe hand injury 5 weeks ago. During an OT session, the client reports that family responsibilities make it impossible to complete the prescribed exercise and splinting program. What action should the OTR take in response to this comment in order to promote the client's successful participation in the home program?

    A. Determine a home program that closely aligns with typical performance patterns.

    B. Analyze a 24-hour log to determine time management issues the client is experiencing.

    C. Advise the client to make the home program the highest priority for the short term.

    D. Suggest transition to a compensatory approach for dealing with residual deficits.

86. A client in an outpatient setting sustained a frontal lobe TBI 2 months ago. The client has good motor control, but has residual problems with executive functioning. One of the client's goals is to be independent with homemaking tasks. During a meal preparation session the client cooks a meal, but makes no attempt to clean the cooking utensils and dishes or put the food items away after completing the cooking task. Which area of executive function appears to be **MOST** affected by the TBI as evidenced by this behavior?

    A. Emergent awareness

    B. Selective attention

    C. Episodic memory

    D. Environmental gnosia

87. A patient with a borderline personality disorder was admitted to an inpatient facility 4 days ago secondary to an exacerbation of suicidal and self-mutilating behavior. The patient's condition is now stable and the patient is functioning at Allen Cognitive Level 5 (Exploratory Actions). The patient reports being overwhelmed by a new personal relationship, experiencing job dissatisfaction, and feeling a lack of control in most daily situations. Which intervention would be **MOST BENEFICIAL** for addressing problems in performance skills and patterns secondary to the concurrent symptoms?

    A. Coping skills groups that address a variety of adaptive strategies

    B. One-on-one sessions to encourage the patient to contract for safety

    C. Daily self-care sessions that focus on structured BADL

    D. Structured one-step craft activities to promote successful outcomes

88. An OTR is preparing for an **INITIAL** intervention session with an inpatient who is in the acute manic phase of bipolar disorder. Which general strategy should the OTR include as part of this session?

    A. Structure the environment to encourage creativity and self-expression.

    B. Minimize distractions in the environment during task performance.

    C. Ensure the patient is aware of the influence of mania on participation.

    D. Provide the patient with an opportunity to select an activity of interest.

89. An OTR is providing recommendations to the caregiver of a client who has moderately severe cognitive decline secondary to Alzheimer's disease. The caregiver reports the client wanders throughout the home at night trying to find the bathroom. On several occasions the client has walked out the front door of the home thinking it was the door leading into the bathroom. Which environmental adaptation should the OTR recommend to the caregiver based on this report?

    A. Use movement sensitive audio-visual assistive technology.

    B. Place a commode chair in the client's bedroom.

    C. Install a video monitor in several locations in the house.

    D. Keep hallway and bedroom lights on at night.

The following multiple-choice items are samples related to Domain 4:

> **Manage and direct occupational therapy services to promote quality in practice.**

90. After becoming initially certified as an OTR, an individual worked in an outpatient OT clinic for 4 years. After that time, the individual did not work as an OT and has not participated in occupational therapy professional development activities for the past 6 years. The individual wants to resume OT clinical practice. What ethical responsibility does the individual have prior to obtaining a job in an outpatient setting?

    A. Identify professional development units that can be carried over from the previous job.

    B. Volunteer as an OT in a clinical setting to establish service competence.

    C. Create an effective learning plan related to skills needed for the desired practice setting.

    D. Submit an application to renew national certification as an OTR.

91. An OTR is reviewing a research article investigating the role of peer support among members living in a retirement community. Data collection methods included observation, note – taking and semi-structured interviews conducted with members over a 6-month period. Constant comparison and open coding were undertaken to categorize core concepts. A conceptual model identifying 5 tiers of peer support was constructed based on members' experience. Which type of qualitative research design does this investigation represent?

    A. Grounded theory study

    B. Participatory action research

    C. Critical theory study

    D. Phenomenological study

92. An OTR working in a pediatric hospital-based clinic wants to begin using a newly developed listening device as part of the OT intervention for children diagnosed with autism. What information is **MOST IMPORTANT** for the OTR to determine prior to using this device with these children?

    A. Outline a standard protocol to use with each child who will use the device.

    B. Identify the clinical practice guidelines and evidence related to using the device.

    C. Develop a plan to monitor the effectiveness of the new intervention.

    D. Determine if third-party payers reimburse the device as a therapeutic modality.

93. A patient who has global aphasia and flaccid hemiplegia secondary to a CVA has been participating in OT. During an employee safety inservice, a customer service employee, who is a distant relative of this patient, asks the OTR about the patient's progress in OT. Which statement represents an appropriate response for the OTR to provide to this inquiry?

    A. "Based on the recent evaluation, the patient has a long way to go."

    B. "I can't talk about the patient without the patient's approval."

    C. "The patient seems to be satisfied with the overall progress."

    D. "I think the patient will have a difficult time returning home."

94. A rheumatologist has prescribed bilateral nighttime resting hand splints for a child who has early stage juvenile rheumatoid arthritis. The parents ask the OTR who works at the child's school to fabricate the splints. Despite having this disease, the child is functioning at grade-level and is not on the OT caseload. What action should the OTR take in response to the parents' request?

    A. Schedule a time after school hours to fabricate the splints for the child.

    B. Initiate an IEP indicating the child's needs for school-based OT.

    C. Inform the parents to schedule an appointment at an outpatient OT clinic.

    D. Provide the parents with catalog information for ordering pre-fabricated splints.

95. An OTR wants to measure the effectiveness of a leisure education program for clients who attend an outpatient chemical dependency unit. What method should the OTR use to obtain a valid measure of the program's effectiveness?

    A. Track the number of clients referred to the program with the number of clients who complete the program.

    B. Compare a measurement of client leisure involvement at the start of the program with leisure involvement upon completion of the program.

    C. Administer a questionnaire about the perceived importance of leisure activities to clients who complete the program.

    D. Monitor the frequency of client attendance and level of participation during each session of the program.

96. An OTR working in a skilled nursing facility frequently teaches residents how to use adaptive devices during BADL. The OTR wants to evaluate if the instruction methods and devices are effective in helping to improve the residents' functional performance. Which method would be **MOST EFFECTIVE** to use for gathering this information?

    A. Note the number of times the residents bring the devices to BADL sessions.

    B. Ask the residents how often during the week they use the devices for BADL.

    C. Have the residents demonstrate the use of the devices during a session.

    D. Track how many times the residents spontaneously use the devices during BADL.

97. A client sustained a hand injury 8 weeks ago and has been participating in an outpatient OT program several times a week for the past 3 weeks. The OTR has just fabricated a dynamic splint to correct a PIP joint contracture. What information is **MOST IMPORTANT** to include in the contact note for this visit?

    A. Results of a sensory evaluation of the affected hand

    B. Goniometric measurements of the affected hand

    C. Thickness and type of material used for the splint

    D. Splint construction methods and care instructions

98. A third-party payer has denied reimbursement of pre-authorized occupational therapy services based on "insufficient information to substantiate payment". The OTR is writing a letter to appeal the denial. What type of client-related information is **MOST IMPORTANT** to include to increase the likelihood of reimbursement?

    A. Outline of functional tasks used during each intervention session

    B. Summary of progress based on functional goals and medical necessity

    C. Annotated reference list indicating evidence-based best practice guidelines

    D. Rate of progress compared to other clients who have the same diagnosis

99. An inpatient in a Medicare-funded rehabilitation facility recently had transtibial amputations of both legs. The patient participates in 3 hours of therapy per day and is currently scheduled for discharge in 2 weeks. During the weekly interprofessional meeting the OTR reports the patient has met the OT intervention goals. The physical therapist reports the patient will continue to require physical therapy 2 hours per day until discharge from the facility in 2 weeks. The prosthetist will also be working with the patient during this time. What action should the OTR take based on the meeting reports?

    A. Complete a discharge summary and discontinue the patient from OT services.

    B. Determine if there are any other activities in which the patient would like to participate.

    C. Schedule the patient for at least one hour of OT per day to meet the 3-hour therapy rule.

    D. Continue to schedule OT sessions to maintain the progress the patient has made thus far.

100. An OTR has completed the initial evaluation of an inpatient who has cancer. The OTR plans to work with the patient on a daily basis prior to the patient's planned discharge to home in one week. What information is **MOST IMPORTANT** to include in the initial evaluation report?

    A. Summary data as it relates to the occupational profile

    B. Details about interventions for promoting goal attainment

    C. Descriptions of community support services available

    D. Recommendations for post-discharge OT services

SECTION 6:

Answers, Rationales, and References

Answer Key for the OTR Study Guide M-C Sample Items

Item #	Key
1	B
2	A
3	D
4	D
5	B
6	D
7	A
8	D
9	C
10	A
11	A
12	C
13	A
14	A
15	B
16	B
17	A
18	D
19	B
20	A
21	C
22	D
23	B
24	B
25	B
26	C
27	C
28	D
29	A
30	D

Item #	Key
31	B
32	A
33	D
34	B
35	B
36	A
37	B
38	C
39	C
40	A
41	B
42	C
43	B
44	D
45	D
46	C
47	C
48	A
49	C
50	D
51	D
52	A
53	B
54	C
55	A
56	D
57	D
58	A
59	B
60	A
61	B
62	C
63	D
64	B
65	B

Item #	Key
66	C
67	B
68	A
69	A
70	B
71	D
72	D
73	A
74	C
75	A
76	A
77	A
78	B
79	C
80	C
81	A
82	C
83	B
84	C
85	A
86	A
87	A
88	B
89	A
90	C
91	A
92	B
93	B
94	C
95	B
96	D
97	B
98	B
99	A
100	A

Multiple-Choice Answers, Rationales, and References

1. Correct Answer: B

This skill requires a complex integration of visual and somatosensory systems that typically develops by the third year of age.

Incorrect Answers:

A, C, D. These self-dressing skills typically develop prior to age 3.

Reference: Case-Smith, J., O'Brien, J. (2010). *Occupational Therapy for Children* (6th ed.). St. Louis, MO: Elsevier Mosby. Page 501.

2. Correct Answer: A

This movement pattern indicates the presence of the symmetrical tonic neck reflex (STNR).

Incorrect Answers:

B, C, D. These movement patterns are not consistent with the STNR.

Reference: Pendleton, H. M., Schultz-Krohn, W. (eds). (2013). *Pedretti's Occupational Therapy: Practice Skills for Physical Dysfunction* (7th ed.). St. Louis, MO: Elsevier Mosby. Pages 474-476.

3. Correct Answer: D

A patient functioning at this level has localized responses to some stimuli. It is important to establish an objective baseline of responsiveness.

Incorrect Answers:

A, B, C. These are not appropriate for a patient who is functioning at Level III (Localized response).

Reference: Pendleton, H. M., Schultz-Krohn, W. (eds). (2013). *Pedretti's Occupational Therapy: Practice Skills for Physical Dysfunction* (7th ed.). St. Louis: Elsevier Mosby. Pages 888-889, 898.

4. Correct Answer: D

Clients who have a complete C_6 spinal cord injury **TYPICALLY** have innervation of the radial wrist extensors. This allows the use of a tenodesis grasp to attain a higher level of functional independence.

Incorrect Answers:

A. Finger and thumb flexors are innervated at the C_7 level.

B. Elbow extension is innervated at the C_7 level and is not present in a complete C_6 spinal cord injury.

C. Trunk control for side bending is absent at the C_5-C_6 level.

Reference: Pendleton, H. M., Schultz-Krohn, W. (eds). (2013). *Pedretti's Occupational Therapy: Practice Skills for Physical Dysfunction* (7th ed.). St. Louis, MO: Elsevier Mosby. Pages 964-966, 969.

5. *Correct Answer: B*

   The client's clinical symptoms are indicative of a median nerve injury. Sensory distribution for the median nerve is to the volar surface of the thumb, index, long, and radial half of the ring fingers.

   Incorrect Answers:

   A, C, D. These are not the typical sensory distributions for the median nerve.

   Reference: Pendleton, H. M., Schultz-Krohn, W. (eds). (2013). *Pedretti's Occupational Therapy: Practice Skills for Physical Dysfunction* (7th ed.). St. Louis, MO: Elsevier Mosby. Pages 1045, 1051-1052.

6. *Correct Answer: D*

   Occupational profiles provide information about the client's priorities. This leads to a more individualized approach to evaluation and intervention planning.

   Incorrect Answers:

   A, B, C. These may be helpful during the evaluation process, but only after completion of a comprehensive occupational profile.

   Reference: Pendleton, H. M., Schultz-Krohn, W. (eds). (2013). *Pedretti's Occupational Therapy: Practice Skills for Physical Dysfunction* (7th ed.). St. Louis, MO: Elsevier Mosby. Pages 938-939.

7. *Correct Answer: A*

   This is a survey used as a measure of general health and well-being. It has been used in medical outcomes studies and is sensitive to change in health status.

   Incorrect Answers:

   B. This is an evaluation of basic living skills and does not measure quality of life.

   C. This reflects the functional status of hospital patients. It is not a measure of quality of life.

   D. This is an evaluation for assessing severity of a disability and does not measure quality of life.

   Reference: Asher, I. E. (2007). *Occupational Therapy Assessment Tool: An Annotated Index.* (3rd ed.). Bethesda, MD: AOTA Press. Pages 64, 80, 102, 224.

8. *Correct Answer: D*

   This fosters collaboration between the client and OTR for developing a meaningful client-centered intervention plan. It can be used to measure change in a client's self-perception of occupational performance over time.

   Incorrect Answers:

   A. This is an evaluation of basic living skills and does not address the client's priorities.

   B. This reflects the functional status of hospital patients and does not address the client's priorities.

   C. This helps to identify roles significant to the client and the motivation to engage in the tasks necessary for those roles.

   Reference: Asher, I. E. (2007). *Occupational Therapy Assessment Tool: An Annotated Index.* (3rd ed.). Bethesda, MD: AOTA Press. Pages 33, 80, 102, 627.

9. *Correct Answer: C*

Volumetric measurement procedures are standardized and would produce the **MOST RELIABLE** results for measuring hand edema for clients with this diagnosis.

Incorrect Answers:

A. This may be a useful screening tool, but inconsistency in tension placed on the tape during the measuring procedures makes this a less reliable option.

B, D. These can be useful for monitoring edema, but typically the procedures for each are not completed using standardized methods.

Reference: Pendleton, H. M., Schultz-Krohn, W. (eds). (2013). *Pedretti's Occupational Therapy: Practice Skills for Physical Dysfunction* (7th ed.). St. Louis: Elsevier Mosby. Pages 1046-1047.

Gillen, G. (2011). *Stroke Rehabilitation: A Function-Based Approach* (3rd ed.). St. Louis, MO: Elsevier Mosby. Page 311.

10. *Correct Answer: A*

Since the patient has intact memory, the behavior suggests topographical disorientation. The test for this is typically a functional test. Contributing visual perceptual deficits should also be considered.

Incorrect Answers:

B, C, D. The client's behaviors are not consistent with deficits in these areas.

Reference: Gillen, G. (2011). *Stroke Rehabilitation: A Function-Based Approach* (3rd ed.). St. Louis, MO: Elsevier Mosby. Pages 430-431, 475, 521.

Pendleton, H. M., Schultz-Krohn, W. (eds). (2013). *Pedretti's Occupational Therapy: Practice Skills for Physical Dysfunction* (7th ed.). St. Louis, MO: Elsevier Mosby. Pages 866-867.

11. *Correct Answer: A*

An understanding of the contexts that impact a child's performance is critical to effective intervention planning.

Incorrect Answers:

B, C, D. This information is helpful but is not a critical component for OT intervention planning.

Reference: Case-Smith, J., O'Brien, J. (2010). *Occupational Therapy for Children* (6th ed.). St. Louis, MO: Elsevier Mosby. Pages 3-5, 193-194.

12. *Correct Answer: C*

Identifying routines and habits is an essential element for reestablishing a patient's occupational performance during this task.

Incorrect Answers:

A, B, D. These can be done after determining a patient's typical routines and habits.

Reference: Pendleton, H. M., Schultz-Krohn, W. (eds). (2013). *Pedretti's Occupational Therapy: Practice Skills for Physical Dysfunction* (7th ed.). St. Louis, MO: Elsevier Mosby. Pages 8-9, 162.

13. *Correct Answer: A*

This answer supports a client-centered, collaborative approach.

Incorrect Answers:

B. Assistive devices may be helpful for increasing independence during ADL, but are not essential for the patient to use. The OTR must emphasize the importance of adhering to specific movement precautions and determine alternative options the patient can use to adhere to these precautions.

C. Using assistive devices may help with occupational performance but they do not necessarily speed up the healing process.

D. The OTR should talk with the patient and spouse prior to documenting an impression or contacting a care coordinator.

Reference: Pendleton, H. M., Schultz-Krohn, W. (eds). (2013). *Pedretti's Occupational Therapy: Practice Skills for Physical Dysfunction* (7th ed.). St. Louis, MO: Elsevier Mosby. Pages 37-38, 101-102, 1083-1086.

14. *Correct Answer: A*

The OTR should consult with the physician, as these may be indicative of clinical depression.

Incorrect Answers:

B. The OTR should not rely on the client to initiate the appointment.

C, D. These may be considered after consulting with the physician.

Reference: Pendleton, H. M., Schultz-Krohn, W. (eds). (2013). *Pedretti's Occupational Therapy: Practice Skills for Physical Dysfunction* (7th ed.). St. Louis, MO: Elsevier Mosby. Pages 875-876.

15. *Correct Answer: B*

Moving from supine to sitting may result in an excessive decrease in blood pressure that reduces blood flow to the brain and results in lightheadedness.

Incorrect Answers:

A, C, D. These are not symptoms directly associated with orthostatic hypotension.

Reference: Pendleton, H. M., Schultz-Krohn, W. (eds). (2013). *Pedretti's Occupational Therapy: Practice Skills for Physical Dysfunction* (7th ed.). St. Louis, MO: Elsevier Mosby. Page 960.

16. *Correct Answer: B*

The patient's physiologic response to activity must be monitored during this early phase of cardiac rehabilitation.

Incorrect Answers:

A, D. These may be included during phase I but are not **ESSENTIAL** during the initial session.

C. Isometric and exertion activities such as those required for strength testing are contraindicated at this phase of rehabilitation.

Reference: Pendleton, H. M., Schultz-Krohn, W. (eds). (2013). *Pedretti's Occupational Therapy: Practice Skills for Physical Dysfunction* (7th ed.). St. Louis, MO: Elsevier Mosby. Pages 1202-1203.

17. *Correct Answer: A*

Ecology of human performance (EHP) model focuses on tasks that acquire meaning through the person-environment interaction. Modifying the client's home environment will enhance the client's well-being and quality of life in that environment.

Incorrect Answers:

B, C, D. These do not specifically support the EHP approach.

Reference: Pendleton, H. M., Schultz-Krohn, W. (eds). (2013). *Pedretti's Occupational Therapy: Practice Skills for Physical Dysfunction* (7th ed.). St. Louis: Elsevier Mosby. Page 39.

18. *Correct Answer: D*

This is an evidence-based functional approach for promoting use of a hemiparetic upper extremity.

Incorrect Answers:

A. This is a bottom-up approach based on a neurophysiological model.

B. This uses a bottom-up approach that aims to inhibit abnormal reflex mechanisms to facilitate function. Evidence related to the efficacy of this approach is controversial.

C. This uses a top-down approach of adapting a client's environment to compensate for symptoms.

Reference: Pendleton, H. M., Schultz-Krohn, W. (eds). (2013). *Pedretti's Occupational Therapy: Practice Skills for Physical Dysfunction* (7th ed.). St. Louis, MO: Elsevier Mosby. Pages 833-838.

19. *Correct Answer: B*

The adaptive approach capitalizes on the client's abilities. This top-down approach aims to facilitate functional performance through compensatory techniques.

Incorrect Answers:

A, C, D. These are examples of a restorative approach.

Reference: Pendleton, H. M., Schultz-Krohn, W. (eds). (2013). *Pedretti's Occupational Therapy: Practice Skills for Physical Dysfunction* (7th ed.). St. Louis: Elsevier Mosby. Pages 124-125.

Zoltan, B. (2007). *Vision, Perception, and Cognition: A Manual for the Evaluation and Treatment of the Adult with Acquired Brain Injury* (4th ed.). Thorofare, NJ: SLACK. Inc. Pages 4-5, 100-103.

20. *Correct Answer: A*

This represents a top-down approach because it focuses on a strategy the client can use in everyday life.

Incorrect Answers:

B, C, D. These are bottom-up restorative approaches.

Reference: Pendleton, H. M., Schultz-Krohn, W. (eds). (2013). *Pedretti's Occupational Therapy: Practice Skills for Physical Dysfunction* (7th ed.). St. Louis: Elsevier Mosby. Page 853.

Gillen, G. (2011). *Stroke Rehabilitation: A Function-Based Approach* (3rd ed.). St. Louis, MO: Elsevier Mosby. Page 554.

21. *Correct Answer: C*

The concept of lifestyle modification in the area of weight management focuses on healthy behavioral changes based on clients' occupational performance patterns.

Incorrect Answers:

A, B, D. These options do not offer a comprehensive approach for facilitating behavioral changes based on clients' occupational performance patterns.

Reference: Scaffa, M. E., Reitz S. M., Pizzi M. A. (2010). *Occupational Therapy in the Promotion of Health and Wellness*. Philadelphia, PA: F. A. Davis Company. Pages 270-271.

22. *Correct Answer: D*

Using this approach allows the patient to learn adaptive strategies, reestablish routines, and learn to function in a variety of contexts.

Incorrect Answers:

A, B, C. These approaches might be incorporated as part of the intervention plan but would not be the **PRIMARY** approach for promoting progress to the patient's homemaking goal.

Reference: Radomski, M. V., Trombly-Latham, C. (2008). *Occupational Therapy for Physical Dysfunction* (6th ed.). Baltimore, MD: Wolters Kluwer, Lippincott, Williams & Wilkins. Pages 55-56, 1175, 1195.

Pendleton, H. M., Schultz-Krohn, W. (eds). (2013). *Pedretti's Occupational Therapy: Practice Skills for Physical Dysfunction* (7th ed.). St. Louis, MO: Elsevier Mosby. Pages 1045, 1051-1052, 964-968.

23. *Correct Answer: B*

Figure-ground perception is the ability to distinguish foreground from background. A student who has figure-ground deficits would have difficulty finding a specific size or shape bead in a bag of beads.

Incorrect Answers:

A, C, D. Figure-ground deficits would not be as evident during these activities.

Reference: Zoltan, B. (2007). *Vision, Perception, and Cognition: A Manual for the Evaluation and Treatment of the Adult with Acquired Brain Injury* (4th ed.). Thorofare, NJ: SLACK. Inc. Pages 155-159.

Case-Smith, J., O'Brien, J. (2010). *Occupational Therapy for Children* (6th ed.). St. Louis, MO: Elsevier Mosby. Page 377.

24. *Correct Answer:* B

The radial nerve is commonly injured with a fracture of the humerus. This results in weak or absent wrist and finger extensors. The OTR should contact the physician to confirm this diagnosis and to clarify the consult before proceeding with rehabilitation for the hand.

Incorrect Answers:

A. This is not indicated in the presence of radial nerve palsy.

C. These may be appropriate after determining if a radial nerve palsy is present and upon clarification of the therapy consult.

D. A comprehensive manual muscle test is not indicated in the presence of a healing fracture.

Reference: Burke, S., Higgins, J., M. Clinton, M., Saunders, R., Valdata, L. (2006). *Hand and Upper Extremity Rehabilitation: A Practical Guide* (3rd ed.). St. Louis, MO: Elsevier Churchill Livingstone. Page 377.

25. *Correct Answer:* B

Ulnar nerve palsy at the wrist impairs the hypothenar muscles and first dorsal interosseous muscle resulting in the difficulty performing a "key" or lateral pinch.

Incorrect Answers:

A. Carrying a briefcase requires a hook grasp which is not affected by a low ulnar nerve injury.

C. This would be less evident when using the index finger to input numbers in a calculator. The lumbrical muscles flex the index finger MCP joint and are innervated by the median nerve.

D. Holding coins in the palm of the hand is not reliant upon an intact ulnar nerve.

Reference: Pendleton, H. M., Schultz-Krohn, W. (eds). (2013). *Pedretti's Occupational Therapy: Practice Skills for Physical Dysfunction* (7th ed.). St. Louis, MO: Elsevier Mosby. Pages 1043-1044, 1052-1053.

26. *Correct Answer:* C

Patients with this muscle strength have low endurance and fatigue quickly. An analysis of the components (e.g., weight shift, dynamic balance, movement against gravity) of each option presented indicates this option is physically more demanding than the other three options.

Incorrect Answers:

A, B, D. These tasks are not as physically demanding as option "C". These tasks would be easier for the patient to accomplish while seated.

Reference: Pendleton, H. M., Schultz-Krohn, W. (eds). (2013). *Pedretti's Occupational Therapy: Practice Skills for Physical Dysfunction* (7th ed.). St. Louis, MO: Elsevier Mosby. Pages 532, 535.

27. *Correct Answer:* C

The assessment should take place in the environment where the patient will typically complete this task. While an inpatient, this is in the bathroom of the patient's room.

Incorrect Answers:

A, B, D. These are not optimal environments for obtaining information about the patient's typical grooming and hygiene routines.

Reference: Pendleton, H. M., Schultz-Krohn, W. (eds). (2013). *Pedretti's Occupational Therapy: Practice Skills for Physical Dysfunction* (7th ed.). St. Louis: Elsevier Mosby. Pages 162-163.

Radomski, M. V., Trombly-Latham, C. (2008). *Occupational Therapy for Physical Dysfunction* (6th ed.). Baltimore, MD: Wolters Kluwer, Lippincott, Williams & Wilkins. Pages 80-82.

28. *Correct Answer:* D

OT goals and objectives in school-based settings support students' academic and functional abilities. Providing services in the natural classroom environment during typical routines would increase the likelihood for carry-over and consistency.

Incorrect Answers:

A, B, C. It may be helpful to occasionally provide the student with an opportunity to practice a particular skill in these environments. However, it would not be as effective for the majority of the intervention sessions.

Reference: Case-Smith, J., O'Brien, J. (2010). *Occupational Therapy for Children* (6th ed.). St. Louis, MO: Elsevier Mosby. Pages 730-731.

29. *Correct Answer:* A

The patient would benefit from learning self-management techniques. One-on-one intervention sessions in the patient's room would be most conducive for promoting initial progress toward the goals. As progress is made, session contexts should be graded to reflect real-life situations.

Incorrect Answers:

B, C, D. These environments would not be conducive for supporting the patient's participation during the initial intervention.

Reference: Cara, E., MacRae, A. (2013). *Psychosocial Occupational Therapy: An Evolving Practice* (3rd ed.). New York, NY: Delmar: Cengage Learning. Pages 280-287.

30. *Correct Answer:* D

Limitations in active ROM, in the presence of full passive ROM, indicate weakness or a lack of power generated by the muscle or muscle group.

Incorrect Answers:

A. These are associated with ALS but would not cause this ROM discrepancy.

B, C. Active and passive ROM would be similarly impacted.

Reference: Pendleton, H. M., Schultz-Krohn, W. (eds). (2013). *Pedretti's Occupational Therapy: Practice Skills for Physical Dysfunction* (7th ed.). St. Louis: Elsevier Mosby. Pages 533-534, 918-921.

31. *Correct Answer: B*

   The percentile score is the percentage of subjects that score at or below a particular raw score.

   Incorrect Answers:

   A, C, D. These are not accurate statements based on the definition of a percentile score.

   Reference: Case-Smith, J., O'Brien, J. (2010). *Occupational Therapy for Children* (6th ed.). St. Louis, MO: Elsevier Mosby. Page 229.

32. *Correct Answer: A*

   The brachioradialis, innervated by the radial nerve, is substituting for weak biceps. This results in movement of the forearm into a midposition when attempting to actively flex the elbow against gravity.

   Incorrect Answers:

   B. The OTR does not have enough information to make this conclusion.

   C. The forearm would fully pronate if substitution patterns were associated with this muscle.

   D. This is not an appropriate testing position for this muscle.

   Reference: Pendleton, H. M., Schultz-Krohn, W. (eds). (2013). *Pedretti's Occupational Therapy: Practice Skills for Physical Dysfunction* (7th ed.). St. Louis, MO: Elsevier Mosby. Page 548.

33. *Correct Answer: D*

   Premotor perseveration results in repetition of movements and difficulty transitioning from one aspect of an activity to another.

   Incorrect Answers:

   A, B, C. The patient's actions during the dressing task are not consistent with these neurobehavioral deficits.

   Reference: Gillen, G. (2011). *Stroke Rehabilitation: A Function-Based Approach* (3rd ed.). St. Louis, MO: Elsevier Mosby. Page 311.

34. *Correct Answer: B*

   The purpose of a criterion-referenced test is to assess the child's performance against a specific criterion or measure, rather than comparing performance to same-age peers. The OTR can use results of criterion-referenced tests to identify specific tasks to use as the focus of intervention.

   Incorrect Answers:

   A, C, D. These are typically associated with normative-referenced tests.

   Reference: Case-Smith, J., O'Brien, J. (2010). *Occupational Therapy for Children* (6th ed.). St. Louis, MO: Elsevier Mosby. Page 224.

35. *Correct Answer: B*

The OTR should complete a re-evaluation prior to discussing other options with the interprofessional team or writing the discharge summary.

Incorrect Answers:

A, C, D. These are not the **INITIAL** actions the OTR should take based on the information provided.

Reference: Pendleton, H. M., Schultz-Krohn, W. (eds). (2013). *Pedretti's Occupational Therapy: Practice Skills for Physical Dysfunction* (7th ed.). St. Louis, MO: Elsevier Mosby. Pages 124, 129.

36. *Correct Answer: A*

The employer is required to provide reasonable accommodations for individuals who have a disability that substantially limit major life activities. Changing a job schedule is considered a reasonable accommodation for this client's job.

Incorrect Answers:

B. Altering essential job tasks is not considered a reasonable accommodation.

C. The employer is not obligated to provide this equipment.

D. These major architectural modifications are not considered reasonable accommodations.

Reference: Pendleton, H. M., Schultz-Krohn, W. (eds). (2013). *Pedretti's Occupational Therapy: Practice Skills for Physical Dysfunction* (7th ed.). St. Louis, MO: Elsevier Mosby. Pages 387-389.

37. *Correct Answer: B*

This method provides the broadest amount of information that is appropriate for this audience.

Incorrect Answers:

A. This information presents a narrow focus and would be more appropriate for an audience of health care team members.

C. This does not address the diverse issues that the group as a whole may have. There are potential health information disclosure issues associated with this presentation method.

D. Generic exercise protocols may not meet individual needs and may be contraindicated for some individuals.

Reference: Fazio, L. (2008) *Developing Occupation-Centered Programming for the Community: A Workbook for Students and Professionals* (2nd Ed.). Upper Saddle River, NJ: Prentice Hall. Pages 363-364.

38. *Correct Answer: C*

    Since the client self-referred to this class, the OTR must have a consult to fabricate the splints. Scheduling an appointment with the rheumatologist would allow the physician to evaluate the client's current condition.

    Incorrect Answers:

    A. A physician referral is typically required for reimbursement of services from insurance companies.

    B. This may be considered after consulting with the physician.

    D. The OTR should not complete a comprehensive evaluation until after receiving a consult.

    Reference: Pendleton, H. M., Schultz-Krohn, W. (eds). (2013). *Pedretti's Occupational Therapy: Practice Skills for Physical Dysfunction* (7th ed.). St. Louis, MO: Elsevier Mosby. Page 30.

39. *Correct Answer: C*

    The primary purpose of an interprofessional team approach is to make collaborative decisions and coordinate patient care. Presenting information about the patient's current abilities enables other team members to reinforce these skills during functional tasks (e.g., properly positioning the patient and providing appropriate assistive devices during meals)

    Incorrect Answers:

    A. These are important to observe, but not important to report at a care coordination meeting.

    B. Specific techniques do not need to be reported at a care coordination meeting.

    D. Typically, patients who have dysphagia are provided with a special diet menu consisting of safe food options.

    Reference: Pendleton, H. M., Schultz-Krohn, W. (eds). (2013). *Pedretti's Occupational Therapy: Practice Skills for Physical Dysfunction* (7th ed.). St. Louis, MO: Elsevier Mosby. Pages 698-699.

40. *Correct Answer: A*

    This is a screening for determining eye dominance.

    Incorrect Answers:

    B, C, D. More information about the client's vision is needed to make these conclusions.

    Reference: Warren, M., Barstow, E. (2011). *Occupational Therapy Interventions for Adults with Low Vision*. Bethesda, MD: AOTA Press. Page 119.

41. Correct Answer: B

The acquisition of practical life management skills is essential for enabling the client to develop a sense of control and autonomy for supporting participation in meaningful occupations.

Incorrect Answers:

A. Moving into an apartment with a supportive friend, without establishing basic life management skills, leaves the client at risk for maladaptive behaviors and other stressors.

C. Leisure activities with social acquaintances may not be effective if the social network includes individuals who are substance users.

D. The stem does not identify work stress as a current issue for this client.

Reference: Boyt-Schell, B. B., Gillen, G., Scaffa, M. E. (2014). *Willard & Spackman's Occupational Therapy* (12th ed.). Baltimore, MD: Wolters Kluwer, Lippincott, Williams & Wilkins. Page 1183.

Cara, E., MacRae, A. (2013). *Psychosocial Occupational Therapy: An Evolving Practice* (3rd ed.). New York, NY: Delmar: Cengage Learning. Pages 841-869.

42. Correct Answer: C

The client's spontaneous use of self-management strategies indicates progress toward the program goals of helping the client learn ways to cope with pain and reduce injury risk during work tasks.

Incorrect Answers:

A, B, D. These are good for the OTR to monitor when working with the client, but they are not the **MOST IMPORTANT** to report to the interprofessional team.

Reference: Pendleton, H. M., Schultz-Krohn, W. (eds). (2013). *Pedretti's Occupational Therapy: Practice Skills for Physical Dysfunction* (7th ed.). St. Louis, MO: Elsevier Mosby. Pages 721, 725, 726.

43. Correct Answer: B

The OTR should formulate the intervention plan based on the outcomes of the initial assessment and in relation to the intended discharge environment. The discharge plans should be reassessed as needed based on the functional progress the patient demonstrates throughout the rehabilitation process.

Incorrect Answers:

A, C. Best practice indicates that the discharge planning process should begin prior to these times.

D. A discharge plan should be implemented for all patients, not just those who have potential to return home.

Reference: Smith-Gabai, H. (2011). *Occupational Therapy in Acute Care.* Bethesda, MD: AOTA Press. Pages 688-689.

44. *Correct Answer:* D

   Use of the assistive devices should be determined based on the patient's needs and priorities. If the patient does not want to use assistive devices, the OTR can still work with the patient to teach energy conservation and other compensatory strategies tailored to predetermined needs and priorities.

   Incorrect Answers:

   A. Equipment selection should be a collaborative process based on the patient's priorities.

   B. The OTR should collaborate with the patient prior to discussing options with the family.

   C. Other compensatory strategies should be explored for improving the patient's occupational performance.

   Reference: Pendleton, H. M., Schultz-Krohn, W. (eds). (2013). *Pedretti's Occupational Therapy: Practice Skills for Physical Dysfunction* (7th ed.). St. Louis, MO: Elsevier Mosby. Pages 196, 985.

45. *Correct Answer:* D

   This is an appropriate intervention for a patient who currently has non-specific, inconsistent, and non-purposeful reactions to stimuli.

   Incorrect Answers:

   A, B, C. These interventions are beneficial for patients who are functioning at higher cognitive levels.

   Reference: Pendleton, H. M., Schultz-Krohn, W. (eds). (2013). *Pedretti's Occupational Therapy: Practice Skills for Physical Dysfunction* (7th ed.). St. Louis, MO: Elsevier Mosby. Pages 888, 898-899.

46. *Correct Answer:* C

   The OTR should provide the client with opportunities to explore work habits and current abilities prior to selecting a specific employment placement.

   Incorrect Answers:

   A. This is a more appropriate option for clients who have intellectual disabilities, significant developmental delay, or a long history of a severe mental illness.

   B, D. These may be options only after the OTR has an understanding of the client's occupational profile and is familiar with the client's work habits. Additionally, it is important for the client to have a realistic perspective of current skills and abilities.

   Reference: Cara, E., MacRae, A. (2013). *Psychosocial Occupational Therapy: An Evolving Practice* (3rd ed.). New York, NY: Delmar: Cengage Learning. Pages 815-819.

47. *Correct Answer: C*

Since a symptom of this disorder includes poor impulse control, providing structure and consistency should be inherent in each treatment session with this adolescent. Additionally, successful experiences help to build self-concept.

Incorrect Answers:

A, B, D. These do not adequately address impulse control or self-concept and are not appropriate during the acute phase of the adolescent's treatment.

Reference: Bonder, B. R. (2010). *Psychopathology and Function* (4th ed.). Thorofare, NJ: SLACK, Inc. Pages 65-66.

48. *Correct Answer: A*

In a Medicare-funded facility, the OTR must prioritize goals based on medical necessity and skilled services needed for function.

Incorrect Answers:

B, C, D. These are not based on function and do not indicate medical necessity or the need for skilled services.

Reference: Gateley, C., Borcherding, S. (2012). *Documentation Manual for Occupational Therapy: Writing SOAP Notes* (3rd ed.). Thorofare, NJ: SLACK, Inc. Pages 13-14, 20.

49. *Correct Answer: C*

During an acute flare up, exercises are important for preserving joint mobility and preventing deformities. Exercises should be completed with caution especially in the presence of painful and swollen joints.

Incorrect Answers:

A, B, D. These exercises may be beneficial after the pain and swelling subside. It is not realistic to include these as a priority for the client to complete by the end of the first week of therapy.

Reference: Pendleton, H. M., Schultz-Krohn, W. (eds). (2013). *Pedretti's Occupational Therapy: Practice Skills for Physical Dysfunction* (7th ed.). St. Louis, MO: Elsevier Mosby. Pages 1020-1024.

50. *Correct Answer: D*

The normal developmental sequence of self-care skills is: feeding, grooming, continence management, transfer skills, toileting, undressing, dressing, and bathing.

Incorrect Answers:

A, B, C. These can be integrated into the intervention plan as indicated by the patient's needs and priorities. But, when following the sequence of normal development, self-feeding would be the **INITIAL** task to start with the patient.

Reference: Pendleton, H. M., Schultz-Krohn, W. (eds). (2013). *Pedretti's Occupational Therapy: Practice Skills for Physical Dysfunction* (7th ed.). St. Louis, MO: Elsevier Mosby. Pages 192-194, 196.

51. *Correct Answer: D*

Deep touch stimuli is typically more tolerable than light touch in the presence of tactile defensiveness.

Incorrect Answers:

A, B. Vestibular input does not necessarily improve tactile defensiveness.

C. Light touch or light stimuli is a common irritant in the presence of tactile defensiveness.

Reference: Case-Smith, J., O'Brien, J. (2010). *Occupational Therapy for Children* (6th ed.). St. Louis, MO: Elsevier Mosby. Pages 346-347.

52. *Correct Answer: A*

An upright orientation helps to decrease directional confusion, provides proprioceptive input for proximal control and promotes a more mature grasp pattern.

Incorrect Answers:

B. Working on a horizontal plane may be confusing for a child who has directional difficulties. This also encourages the use of a palmar grasp.

C. Cutting with adapted scissors encourages a gross opening and closing hand movement. It does not necessarily address the underlying musculoskeletal components required for a mature pencil grasp.

D. Providing hand-over-hand assistance is not an effective use of the sensorimotor approach for this student.

Reference: Case-Smith, J., O'Brien, J. (2010). *Occupational Therapy for Children* (6th ed.). St. Louis, MO: Elsevier Mosby. Pages 567-576.

53. *Correct Answer: B*

These types of contractures respond positively to serial casting and gel sheeting. The child can wear the splint intermittently during the day and all night. Functional use of the hand should be encouraged when the splint is removed.

Incorrect Answers:

A. Increasing the intensity of the exercises may be harmful to the child.

C. It is helpful to provide this information to the caregiver, but it is not the **MOST EFFECTIVE** method for dealing with the contracture.

D. This is not effective for dealing with the contracture.

Reference: Pendleton, H. M., Schultz-Krohn, W. (eds). (2013). *Pedretti's Occupational Therapy: Practice Skills for Physical Dysfunction* (7th ed.). St. Louis, MO: Elsevier Mosby. Pages 1134-1135.

Cooper, C. (2007). *Fundamentals of Hand Therapy: Clinical Reasoning and Treatment Guidelines for Common Diagnoses of the Upper Extremity*. St. Louis, MO: Mosby. Pages 398-399.

54. *Correct Answer: C*

Positioning and postural alignment impact oral motor control. The OTR should evaluate the child's current seating during mealtimes and recommend specific feeding positions and positioning devices.

Incorrect Answers:

A. This method is not effective to use with a child who has oral hypersensitivity.

B. Placing the neck in full forward flexion during feeding may interfere with breathing.

D. These techniques can be completed by the OTR as part of the intervention, but not by the caregiver.

Reference: Case-Smith, J., O'Brien, J. (2010). *Occupational Therapy for Children* (6th ed.). St. Louis, MO: Elsevier Mosby. Pages 458-459.

55. *Correct Answer: A*

Improving postural alignment and stability helps promote oral motor function.

Incorrect Answers:

B, C. These do not provide adequate external support for proper alignment.

D. Postural alignment is too difficult to control in this type of chair.

Reference: Case-Smith, J., O'Brien, J. (2010). *Occupational Therapy for Children* (6th ed.). St. Louis, MO: Elsevier Mosby. Pages 548-459.

56. *Correct Answer: D*

This allows positioning of the trunk posterior to the pelvis and accommodates for the forces of gravity against upright positioning.

Incorrect Answers:

A, B. These are not optimal for engagement in school activities.

C. This does not address the student's intolerance for upright sitting.

Reference: Case-Smith, J., O'Brien, J. (2010). *Occupational Therapy for Children* (6th ed.). St. Louis, MO: Elsevier Mosby. Pages 637-643.

57. *Correct Answer: D*

Using activity analysis methods it is evident that this option provides opportunity for weight bearing with the wrists in extension. This will assist in elongating the soft tissue that is inhibiting motion.

Incorrect Answers:

A, B, C. These may incorporate wrist motion, but they are not as effective for providing soft tissue stretch.

Reference: Pendleton, H. M., Schultz-Krohn, W. (eds). (2013). *Pedretti's Occupational Therapy: Practice Skills for Physical Dysfunction* (7th ed.). St. Louis, MO: Elsevier Mosby. Pages 739-752.

58. *Correct Answer: A*

Axonotmesis results in loss of protective sensation to the affected nerve distribution. This injury does not require surgical intervention and typically resolves within 6 months from initial injury. Since sensation is impaired in the ulnar distribution, it is **MOST IMPORTANT** to teach the client to use visual skills as a compensatory means of protecting the hand from further injury.

Incorrect Answers:

B. This is not indicated for this injury.

C. This can be initiated when Trace (1/5) muscle strength is evident.

D. This can be initiated as indicated when vibratory sensation is perceived.

Reference: Pendleton, H. M., Schultz-Krohn, W. (eds). (2013). *Pedretti's Occupational Therapy: Practice Skills for Physical Dysfunction* (7th ed.). St. Louis, MO: Elsevier Mosby. Pages 578, 1050.

59. *Correct Answer: B*

The OTR should teach the client and caregiver to position the distal end of the client's extremity approximately 3.5 inches (9 cm) above the heart. Elevation to this height allows gravity to assist with hemodynamic fluid transport.

Incorrect Answers:

A. Compression wrapping may cause adverse cyanotic changes in a hemiplegic extremity.

C. Evidence indicates retrograde massage is not as effective as manual edema mobilization or elevation for managing edema.

D. Passive ROM helps to maintain tissue length, but is not a primary means for managing edema.

Reference: Gillen, G. (2011). *Stroke Rehabilitation: A Function-Based Approach* (3rd ed.). St. Louis, MO: Elsevier Mosby. Pages 313-320.

Radomski, M. V., Trombly-Latham, C. (2008). *Occupational Therapy for Physical Dysfunction* (6th ed.). Baltimore, MD: Wolters Kluwer, Lippincott, Williams & Wilkins. Page 1152.

60. *Correct Answer: A*

This is a technique used with clients who have difficulty initiating motion due to rigidity associated with this stage of Parkinson's disease.

Incorrect Answers:

B, C, D. These would not be effective for providing the momentum needed to rise from the bath bench.

Reference: Pendleton, H. M., Schultz-Krohn, W. (eds). (2013). *Pedretti's Occupational Therapy: Practice Skills for Physical Dysfunction* (7th ed.). St. Louis, MO: Elsevier Mosby. Pages 483, 943-945.

61. *Correct Answer:* B

   Using a wheeled cart to transport items from one area of the kitchen to another minimizes stress on smaller finger joints.

   Incorrect Answers:

   A, C, D. These are not consistent with the principles of joint protection.

   Reference: Pendleton, H. M., Schultz-Krohn, W. (eds). (2013). *Pedretti's Occupational Therapy: Practice Skills for Physical Dysfunction* (7th ed.). St. Louis, MO: Elsevier Mosby. Pages 1029-1031.

62. *Correct Answer:* C

   Monitoring symptoms and using appropriate work-rest ratios will minimize the likelihood of becoming physically exhausted.

   Incorrect Answers:

   A. This does not adequately address methods the patient can use to reduce fatigue.

   B, D. These do not take into consideration the patient's typical habits and routines for BADL.

   Reference: Pendleton, H. M., Schultz-Krohn, W. (eds). (2013). *Pedretti's Occupational Therapy: Practice Skills for Physical Dysfunction* (7th ed.). St. Louis, MO: Elsevier Mosby. Pages 936-940.

63. *Correct Answer:* D

   Patients at this level of function have most success during simplified and highly structured tasks. Providing one-step instructions and hand-over-hand assistance supports the patient's participation with the grooming task.

   Incorrect Answers:

   A, B, C. These options may be used as effective intervention techniques as the patient's level of function improves.

   Reference: Radomski, M. V., Trombly-Latham, C. (2008). *Occupational Therapy for Physical Dysfunction* (6th ed.). Baltimore, MD: Wolters Kluwer, Lippincott, Williams & Wilkins. Pages 1059-1060.

64. *Correct Answer:* B

   This is an effective pursed-lip breathing technique for reducing the dyspnea.

   Incorrect Answers:

   A, C. These are not effective techniques for reducing the dyspnea.

   D. Supplemental oxygen is not indicated with an oxygen saturation of 93%.

   Reference: Pendleton, H. M., Schultz-Krohn, W. (eds). (2013). *Pedretti's Occupational Therapy: Practice Skills for Physical Dysfunction* (7th ed.). St. Louis, MO: Elsevier Mosby. Pages 1207-1208.

65. *Correct Answer: B*

   Insidious onset of shoulder restrictions can occur due to disuse and protective posturing. It is **MOST BENEFICIAL** to include ROM exercises of the unaffected joints in the intervention plan.

   Incorrect Answers:

   A. Positioning in a standard pouch sling should be avoided, as they promote disuse and protective posturing.

   C. MCP joint blocking splints are typically not needed during the initial phase of intervention for distal radius fractures.

   D. Using a dry whirlpool modality such as Fluidotherapy® could potentially contaminate the external fixator pin sites.

   Reference: Radomski, M. V., Trombly-Latham, C. (2008). *Occupational Therapy for Physical Dysfunction* (6th ed.). Baltimore, MD: Wolters Kluwer, Lippincott, Williams & Wilkins. Page 1152.

   Cooper, C. (2007). *Fundamentals of Hand Therapy: Clinical Reasoning and Treatment Guidelines for Common Diagnoses of the Upper Extremity*. St. Louis, MO: Elsevier Mosby. Pages 257-259.

66. *Correct Answer: C*

   Edema reduction must be a priority of the intervention.

   Incorrect Answers:

   A, B, D. These interventions do not focus on reducing edema, and may be contraindicated at this stage of the treatment

   Reference: Pendleton, H. M., Schultz-Krohn, W. (eds). (2013). *Pedretti's Occupational Therapy: Practice Skills for Physical Dysfunction* (7th ed.). St. Louis, MO: Elsevier Mosby. Pages 1049, 1059-1060.

67. *Correct Answer: B*

   Heterotopic bone formation results in loss of active ROM of the elbow. Flexion, extension and supination are typically affected.

   Incorrect Answers:

   A. This device is used for patients who have a weak functional grasp.

   C. This device is used for patients who only have use of one upper extremity.

   D. This device is used for patients who have no functional use of the upper extremities.

   Reference: Pendleton, H. M., Schultz-Krohn, W. (eds). (2013). *Pedretti's Occupational Therapy: Practice Skills for Physical Dysfunction* (7th ed.). St. Louis, MO: Elsevier Mosby. Pages 1139, 199.

68. *Correct Answer: A*

   Cerebellar lesions result in ataxia and dysmetria. These assistive devices will help the client stabilize the plate and hold the cup during a meal.

   Incorrect Answers:

   B. A side-cutting fork and a rocker knife are typically used for clients who have unilateral impairment.

   C. These lightweight items are typically recommended for clients who have muscular weakness.

   D. A universal cuff is used to substitute for a weak functional grasp. A mobile arm support (MAS) is used in the presence of proximal arm weakness. The MAS is contraindicated for clients with ataxia.

   Reference: Pendleton, H. M., Schultz-Krohn, W. (eds). (2013). *Pedretti's Occupational Therapy: Practice Skills for Physical Dysfunction* (7th ed.). St. Louis, MO: Elsevier Mosby. Pages 204-206.

69. *Correct Answer: A*

   To increase muscle endurance the number of repetitions must be increased while maintaining the resistance at 50% or less of maximal.

   Incorrect Answers:

   B. This activity will increase speed.

   C, D. These activities promote increased strength.

   Reference: Pendleton, H. M., Schultz-Krohn, W. (eds). (2013). *Pedretti's Occupational Therapy: Practice Skills for Physical Dysfunction* (7th ed.). St. Louis, MO: Elsevier Mosby. Pages 737-738, 741.

70. *Correct Answer: B*

   Using pulleys to passively lift the affected arm overhead increases the risk of shoulder impingement syndrome and upper extremity pain.

   Incorrect Answers:

   A, C, D. These are recommended for managing upper extremity spasticity.

   Reference: Pendleton, H. M., Schultz-Krohn, W. (eds). (2013). *Pedretti's Occupational Therapy: Practice Skills for Physical Dysfunction* (7th ed.). St. Louis, MO: Elsevier Mosby. Pages 871-873.

71. *Correct Answer:* D

Due to the irregular shape of the metacarpal head, the MCP joint collateral ligaments are tight when the MCP joint is in flexion. By positioning the MCP joints between 60°-70° of flexion, the MCP joint collateral ligaments will be taut and the formation of MCP flexion contractures is minimized. Positioning the IP joints in 0°-5° flexion discourages the formation of IP joint flexion contractures caused by shortening of the volar plate, collateral ligaments, and adhesions of the lateral bands.

Incorrect Answers:

A, B, C. The position of the MCP joints in these options does not maintain the optimal length of the MCP joint collateral ligaments. The position of the IP joints also promotes flexion contractures.

Reference: Pendleton, H. M., Schultz-Krohn, W. (eds). (2013). *Pedretti's Occupational Therapy: Practice Skills for Physical Dysfunction* (7th ed.). St. Louis, MO: Elsevier Mosby. Pages 1127-1129.

72. *Correct Answer:* D

A claw-hand deformity is characterized by hyperextension of the fourth and fifth digits and is typically secondary to an ulnar nerve injury. Blocking the fourth and fifth MCP joints in slight flexion allows the extensor digitorum communis tendon to extend the IP joints in the absence of the ulnar innervated intrinsic muscles. The splint will enable the client to have a more functional grasp.

Incorrect Answers:

A, B, C. These splints are not appropriate to use for a claw-hand deformity secondary to an ulnar nerve injury.

Reference: Pendleton, H. M., Schultz-Krohn, W. (eds). (2013). *Pedretti's Occupational Therapy: Practice Skills for Physical Dysfunction* (7th ed.). St. Louis, MO: Elsevier Mosby. Pages 1050- 1053.

Coppard, B. M. & Lohman, H. (2008). *Introduction to Splinting: A Clinical-Reasoning & Problem Solving Approach* (3rd ed.). St. Louis, MO: Elsevier Mosby. Pages 292-293.

73. *Correct Answer:* A

The tub transfer bench provides the patient with the safest method for transferring from/to the wheelchair and bathtub.

Incorrect Answers:

B, C, D. A shower chair or stool does not provide the patient with a safe transfer surface for transferring to either the shower or the tub.

Reference: Pendleton, H. M., Schultz-Krohn, W. (eds). (2013). *Pedretti's Occupational Therapy: Practice Skills for Physical Dysfunction* (7th ed.). St. Louis, MO: Elsevier Mosby. Pages 192-194.

74. *Correct Answer: C*

A mobile arm support attaches to a wheelchair and supports the arm at the elbow allowing the client to use residual upper extremity strength for mobility during functional activities. This device is **CONTRAINDICATED** to use if a client has a significant increase in upper extremity flexor tone or chorea movement patterns.

Incorrect Answers:

A, B, D. Clients who have these diagnoses typically experience proximal upper extremity weakness, but have sufficient ROM and adequate motor control for using a mobile arm support during ADL.

Reference: Pendleton, H. M., Schultz-Krohn, W. (eds). (2013). *Pedretti's Occupational Therapy: Practice Skills for Physical Dysfunction* (7th ed.). St. Louis, MO: Elsevier Mosby. Pages 786-790, 932-936.

75. *Correct Answer: A*

This is recommended for clients who have limited motion for gripping small handles.

Incorrect Answers:

B. This is for clients who have lost the use of one side of the body.

C. This is for clients who have limited active motion of the hand.

D. Decreasing the weight of the utensils will not improve the client's ability to grasp them.

Reference: Pendleton, H. M., Schultz-Krohn, W. (eds). (2013). *Pedretti's Occupational Therapy: Practice Skills for Physical Dysfunction* (7th ed.). St. Louis, MO: Elsevier Mosby. Page 199.

76. *Correct Answer: A*

After positioning the wheelchair and locking the brakes, the client should scoot both hips forward to the edge of the chair. Prior to standing, the client's feet should be positioned firmly on the floor and both knees should be flexed to 90°. This position provides a safe base of support to enable the client to come to standing and then pivot toward the transfer surface.

Incorrect Answers:

B. The client should not come to a standing position until the hips are moved forward to the edge of the wheelchair.

C. The OTR may ask the client to rock back and forth to gain momentum for standing; but only after the hips are forward in the chair and the feet are properly positioned.

D. Placing the feet in this position presents a fall risk to the patient.

Reference: Pendleton, H. M., Schultz-Krohn, W. (eds). (2013). *Pedretti's Occupational Therapy: Practice Skills for Physical Dysfunction* (7th ed.). St. Louis, MO: Elsevier Mosby. Page 255.

77. *Correct Answer:* A

This allows optimal positioning for designated hip precautions.

Incorrect Answers:

B. Clients typically use the arms of a chair to push off during transfers.

C, D. These do not support positioning recommendations and precautions.

Reference: Pendleton, H. M., Schultz-Krohn, W. (eds). (2013). *Pedretti's Occupational Therapy: Practice Skills for Physical Dysfunction* (7th ed.). St. Louis, MO: Elsevier Mosby. Page 1084.

Radomski, M. V., Trombly-Latham, C. (2008). *Occupational Therapy for Physical Dysfunction* (6th ed.). Baltimore, MD: Wolters Kluwer, Lippincott, Williams & Wilkins. Pages 1120-1121.

78. *Correct Answer:* B

Tactile markings will enable the client to monitor the settings on appliances. This will improve kitchen safety especially associated with meal preparations.

Incorrect Answers:

A, C, D. These will not have a significant impact on kitchen safety.

Reference: Pendleton, H. M., Schultz-Krohn, W. (eds). (2013). *Pedretti's Occupational Therapy: Practice Skills for Physical Dysfunction* (7th ed.). St. Louis, MO: Elsevier Mosby. Pages 227-228.

79. *Correct Answer:* C

Modifying the wheelchair by adding a solid seat insert helps to establish and maintain pelvic alignment for improved postural support. Forearm supports provide external support for the weak upper extremities. These modifications aid in reducing postural discomfort and muscular fatigue.

Incorrect Answers:

A. This option does not address ergonomic positioning while the client is seated at the desk.

B. This option may relieve fatigue caused by typing or holding a telephone receiver. It does not address poor postural alignment secondary to sitting for prolonged periods of time in a wheelchair with a sling seat. Proper seating and good postural alignment are paramount for the client's support and comfort.

D. Pelvic alignment and postural support should be addressed first. There is no indication that the client needs a deltoid aid or a split design keyboard.

Reference: Pendleton, H. M., Schultz-Krohn, W. (eds). (2013). *Pedretti's Occupational Therapy: Practice Skills for Physical Dysfunction* (7th ed.). St. Louis, MO: Elsevier Mosby. Pages 248-252, 352-356.

80. *Correct Answer:* C

This option most closely aligns with the client's current habits and routines.

Incorrect Answers:

A, B, D. These require the client to change habits and routines without addressing the need to improve efficiency or make the task easier to complete.

Reference: Pendleton, H. M., Schultz-Krohn, W. (eds). (2013). *Pedretti's Occupational Therapy: Practice Skills for Physical Dysfunction* (7th ed.). St. Louis, MO: Elsevier Mosby. Pages 8-9, 226-227.

81. *Correct Answer:* A

This option aligns with the patient's current functional level and short-term goal to independently bake cookies.

Incorrect Answers:

B, C. These activities require more concentration and focus. The patient would not likely be successful in the completion of these tasks.

D. This task does not support the patient's goal of completing the task independently.

Reference: Pendleton, H. M., Schultz-Krohn, W. (eds). (2013). *Pedretti's Occupational Therapy: Practice Skills for Physical Dysfunction* (7th ed.). St. Louis, MO: Elsevier Mosby. Pages 736-738, 888-889, 893-894.

82. *Correct Answer:* C

To avoid adverse postural reactions, changes to the patient's position should be incremental and gradual. Positioning the patient's upper body in a more upright position, while keeping the legs elevated, reduces the risk of orthostatic hypotension.

Incorrect Answers:

A, B, D. In each of these options, the upright position and dependent leg position increases the risk for orthostatic hypotension.

Reference: Smith-Gabai, H. (2011). *Occupational Therapy in Acute Care*. Bethesda, MD: AOTA Press. Pages 126-127.

Radomski, M. V., Trombly-Latham, C. (2008). *Occupational Therapy for Physical Dysfunction* (6th ed.). Baltimore, MD: Wolters Kluwer, Lippincott, Williams & Wilkins. Page 1176.

83. *Correct Answer:* B

Since the family will be the primary caregivers in the home, it would be **MOST BENEFICIAL** for them to learn how to provide the patient with the stand-by assistance needed for safe functional ambulation.

Incorrect Answers:

A. This is not the role of the caregiver.

C. The patient should use energy conservation techniques during ADL, but for safe transition to the home it is more important for the family caregivers to learn transfer techniques.

D. The patient should be able to complete this task without caregiver assistance.

Reference: Boyt-Schell, B. B., Gillen, G., Scaffa, M. E. (2014). *Willard & Spackman's Occupational Therapy* (12th ed.). Baltimore, MD: Wolters Kluwer, Lippincott, Williams & Wilkins. Pages 645-647.

84. *Correct Answer: C*

In the presence of complex regional pain syndrome (CRPS), vasospasm and vasodilation results in an abnormal persistence of edema. Edema control is important to include in a home program. If edema is not controlled, the protein-rich exudates that cause swelling will result in collagen formation, causing joint stiffness and decrease in functional mobility.

Incorrect Answers:

A. Passive ROM exercises should be avoided in the presence of acute CRPS as they may aggravate the cycle of pain, swelling, and stiffness.

B. Active motion is recommended for preventing joint stiffness, maintaining differential tendon glide, and reducing edema.

D. Including instructions for energy conservation is not critical to intervention for CRPS.

Reference: Pendleton, H. M., Schultz-Krohn, W. (eds). (2013). *Pedretti's Occupational Therapy: Practice Skills for Physical Dysfunction* (7th ed.). St. Louis, MO: Elsevier Mosby. Pages 1062-1063.

85. *Correct Answer: A*

The home program should be contextually relevant and meet the client's needs.

Incorrect Answers:

B, C. These are not effective client-centered strategies.

D. This suggests the client will be unable to regain lost function and must rely on assistive devices.

Reference: Pendleton, H. M., Schultz-Krohn, W. (eds). (2013). *Pedretti's Occupational Therapy: Practice Skills for Physical Dysfunction* (7th ed.). St. Louis, MO: Elsevier Mosby. Pages 160-161.

86. *Correct Answer: A*

This is the ability to recognize and react to situations as they are occurring. = emergent awareness

Incorrect Answers:

B. This involves activating and inhibiting responses based on discrimination of stimulus information. = selective attention

C. This involves memory of a past event. = episodic memory

D. Clients with environmental agnosia get lost in familiar places. = environmental agnosia

Reference: Zoltan, B. (2007). *Vision, Perception, and Cognition: A Manual for the Evaluation and Treatment of the Adult with Acquired Brain Injury* (4th ed.). Thorofare, NJ: SLACK, Inc. Pages 236-238, 244-245.

87. *Correct Answer: A*

Patients functioning at this cognitive level typically are able to use problem solving and inductive reasoning. This type of group provides the patient with opportunities to learn adaptive coping strategies that can be used in a variety of situations relative to the patient's typical performance skills and patterns.

Incorrect Answers:

B. The patient is now medically stable. OT should focus on helping the patient learn adaptive strategies that can be used after discharge.

C. BADL skills are unaffected at this level. However, the patient's ineffective coping skills may lead them to ignore these basic tasks.

D. This type of structured activity is not indicated for higher-functioning patients.

Reference: Bonder, B. R. (2010). *Psychopathology and Function* (4th ed.). Thorofare, NJ: SLACK, Inc. Pages 196-197.

Brown, C., Stoffel, C. (2011). *Occupational Therapy in Mental Health: A Vision for Participation.* Philadelphia, PA: F. A. Davis Company. Pages 143-153.

88. *Correct Answer: B*

It is important to provide a structured environment with minimal distractions during the initial phase of intervention.

Incorrect Answers:

A. This may have negative effects on the patient's ability to complete concrete tasks.

C, D. These do not provide the structure the patient needs during the acute phase of the disorder.

Reference: Cara, E., MacRae, A. (2013). *Psychosocial Occupational Therapy: An Evolving Practice* (3rd ed.). New York, NY: Delmar: Cengage Learning. Pages 231-232, 238.

89. *Correct Answer: A*

Using motion sensitive audio-visual assistive technology is the safest option for promoting a least restrictive and safe home environment. Caregivers will be alerted to the client's movements if the client wanders at night.

Incorrect Answers:

B. The client may still wander through the home without caregiver knowledge.

C. This type of monitor does not have the auditory component to alert the caregiver at night.

D. This is not adequate to ensure that the client remains safe while in the home.

Reference: Pendleton, H. M., Schultz-Krohn, W. (eds). (2013). *Pedretti's Occupational Therapy: Practice Skills for Physical Dysfunction* (7th ed.). St. Louis, MO: Elsevier Mosby. Pages 926-928.

Brown, C., Stoffel, C. (2011). *Occupational Therapy in Mental Health: A Vision for Participation.* Philadelphia, PA: F. A. Davis Company. Pages 234-235.

90. *Correct Answer: C*

> OT practitioners have the ethical responsibility to recognize their current level of professional competence. Creating an effective learning plan related to skills needed for the desired practice setting is a good start in this process.

Incorrect Answers:

> A. These are outdated and cannot be used to meet professional development requirements for certification renewal or licensure.

> B. This individual does not meet the certification renewal or licensure requirements to practice as an OT in a volunteer capacity.

> D. This individual must have proof of current professional development activities prior to submitting these applications.

> **Reference:** Jacobs, K., M. Cormack, G. (eds). (2011). *The Occupational Therapy Manager* (5th ed.). Bethesda, MD: AOTA Press. Pages 485-496.

91. *Correct Answer: A*

> Grounded theory is a research method in which there is continuous comparison between collected data and interpretation resulting in a set of categories and emerging theory.

Incorrect Answers:

> B. Participatory action research is a method by which researchers and those they study enter into a partnership to identify the best way to examine a problem with the aim that the research will make a difference to those who were studied.

> C. Critical theory seeks to understand via reflective inquiry how underlying assumptions can emerge over time against a broader social context.

> D. Phenomenological research typically involves in-depth conversations in which the researcher and informant are fully interactive. Analysis guides decisions on further data collections. The final outcome is generally a theoretical statement often validated by direct quotes from the subjects.

> **Reference:** Kielhofner, G. (2006) *Research in Occupational Therapy: Methods of Inquiry for Enhancing Practice*. F. A. Davis Company. Page 333.

92. *Correct Answer: B*

> This type of appraisal relates to evidence-based practice (EBP) procedures and should be completed prior to using this device or implementing a new clinical procedure related to the use of this device.

Incorrect Answers:

> A, C. These can be developed after determining if the device is safe and appropriate for OT clinical use.

> D. Reimbursements should be considered only after the device is determined safe and appropriate for OT clinical use.

> **Reference:** Jacobs, K., M. Cormack, G. (eds). (2011). *The Occupational Therapy Manager* (5th ed.). Bethesda, MD: AOTA Press. Pages 331-340.

93. *Correct Answer: B*

Even though the co-worker is the patient's relative, there is no evidence that the patient has given signed consent to provide this relative with personal health information. The OTR should advise the co-worker of the need for patient approval.

Incorrect Answers:

A, C, D. These responses violate the patient's confidentiality rights.

Reference: Jacobs, K., M. Cormack, G. (eds). (2011). *The Occupational Therapy Manager* (5th ed.). Bethesda, MD: AOTA Press. Pages 610-611.

94. *Correct Answer: C*

School-based OT must relate to curriculum-based activities. These splints are typically preventive positioning splints for nighttime use. Since this intervention is not directly related to curriculum-based activities and the splints will not be worn during the school day, the OTR should refer the child to an outpatient OT clinic for the splints.

Incorrect Answers:

A. This is not appropriate practice for a school-based OT.

B. There is no need to initiate an IEP since the child is functioning at grade-level.

D. Providing this information to the parents should not be done without the appropriate OT evaluation and splint fitting.

Reference: Case-Smith, J., O'Brien, J. (2010). *Occupational Therapy for Children* (6th ed.). St. Louis, MO: Elsevier Mosby. Pages 716-717.

95. *Correct Answer: B*

This method provides measurable performance-based information for evaluating program effectiveness.

Incorrect Answers:

A, C, D. These options do not provide comparative data against which program objectives can be measured.

Reference: Fazio, L. (2008) *Developing Occupation-Centered Programming for the Community: A Workbook for Students and Professionals* (2nd Ed.). Upper Saddle River, NJ: Prentice Hall. Pages 263-281.

96. *Correct Answer: D*

Tracking spontaneous use of the devices during BADL provides the best indication of transfer of learning and the impact of the device on residents' functional performance.

Incorrect Answers:

A, B, C. These may have an indirect link to functional performance. However, they are not the best indicators of the impact of adaptive devices on the residents' participation in specific BADL tasks.

Reference: Pendleton, H. M., Schultz-Krohn, W. (eds). (2013). *Pedretti's Occupational Therapy: Practice Skills for Physical Dysfunction* (7th ed.). St. Louis, MO: Elsevier Mosby. Page 109.

97. *Correct Answer: B*

Goniometric measurements provide objective baseline information for tracking efficacy of the splint.

Incorrect Answers:

A. It is more important to track changes in ROM to determine the effectiveness of the splint.

C, D. It is not necessary to include this information in the client contact note.

Reference: Coppard, B. M. & Lohman, H. (2008). *Introduction to Splinting: A Clinical-Reasoning & Problem Solving Approach* (3rd ed.). St. Louis, MO: Elsevier Mosby. Pages 48, 108.

Cooper, C. (2007). *Fundamentals of Hand Therapy: Clinical Reasoning and Treatment Guidelines for Common Diagnoses of the Upper Extremity*. St. Louis, MO: Mosby. Pages 278-282.

98. *Correct Answer: B*

The letter of appeal for a pre-authorized visit should include evidence of functional outcomes and medical necessity.

Incorrect Answers:

A, C, D. These do not address the client's functional goals related to the occupational therapy intervention.

Reference: Sladyk, K., Jacobs, K., MacRae N. (2010). *Occupational Therapy Essentials for Clinical Competence*. Thorofare, NJ: SLACK, Inc. Pages 377-382.

99. *Correct Answer: A*

The 3-hour rule is a touchstone the Centers for Medicare and Medicaid use for making an initial finding of medical necessity. The patient can continue to participate in PT for 2 hours per day despite being discharged from OT. Developing new intervention goals is considered fraudulent unless the goals are deemed medically necessary.

Incorrect Answers:

B, C, D. Interventions must be medically necessary and require skilled services.

Reference: Boyt-Schell, B. B., Gillen, G., Scaffa, M. E. (2014). *Willard & Spackman's Occupational Therapy* (12th ed.). Baltimore, MD: Wolters Kluwer, Lippincott, Williams & Wilkins. Pages 1055-1062.

100. *Correct Answer: A*

Initial reports should include evaluation results as they relate to a patient's overall occupational profile.

Incorrect Answers:

B, C, D. These are not essential elements of the initial evaluation report.

Reference: Gateley, C., Borcherding, S. (2012). *Documentation Manual for Occupational Therapy: Writing SOAP Notes* (3rd ed.). Thorofare, NJ: SLACK, Inc. Pages 4, 158-159.

SECTION 7

OTR Multiple-Choice Study Items in Scenario Format

This section contains eight scenarios spanning a range of populations and practice settings. Each scenario has five multiple-choice items linked to an introductory passage (header). The domain area classification, correct answer, rationale for the correct answer, and reference associated with each multiple-choice item are provided is Section 8 of this study guide.

As you approach each scenario, consider what you already know about the subject (Refer to Scenario Formats in Section 4). Reflect on your previous experiences from fieldwork, labs, case studies, and readings. Organize the information presented in the scenario by using the methods presented in Section 4.

After answering each of the scenario-based multiple-choice items, compare your answers to the answer key provided. Flag any items you have scored incorrectly. Read the justification for the correct response, and follow-up using the reference provided as a guide for additional study on the topic.

Scenario A:

An OTR in an <u>outpatient setting</u> is developing an intervention plan for an 18-month old infant with cerebral palsy. The infant has moderate oral-sensory defensiveness and has been receiving nutritive support through a gastrostomy tube since soon after birth. The parents report the infant can only tolerate thickened pureed food due to a hyperactive gag reflex and oral motor delays. The parents' primary goal is to transition the infant to oral feeding.

1A. Which activity demand would have the **MOST** impact on this infant's transition to oral feeding?

A. Infant's ability to interact with others during meals

B. Presence of righting and equilibrium reactions when eating

C. Proficiency for manipulating eating utensils without spillage

D. Trunk stability when sitting in a standard child's highchair

2A. In addition to evaluating client factors that impact oral feeding, what information should the OTR obtain prior to implementing a feeding program for this infant?

A. The parents' specific childrearing beliefs and family routines

B. Ability of the parents to follow a designated home program

C. Signed consent agreeing to accompany infant to all sessions

D. Intervention outcomes from previous service providers

3A. Which technique should the OTR teach the parents to do with the infant between mealtimes as part of a home program for progressing toward the feeding goal?

A. Provide downward pressure on the infant's tongue using a syrup-coated spoon.

B. Rub the infant's gums with light sustained pressure using a moistened washcloth.

C. Apply cold stimulation to the infant's tongue and soft palate using a frozen pacifier.

D. Encourage the infant to explore the mouth using a rubber toy dipped in applesauce.

4A. Which method should the OTR advise the parents to use when positioning the infant for feeding activities?

    A. Hold the infant sideways in the parent's lap resting next to the parent's non-dominant arm.

    B. Sit the infant in a car seat placed on top of the dining table directly in front of the parent.

    C. Have the parent kneel adjacent to the infant placed in a cradle bouncer on the floor.

    D. Place the infant in a beanbag chair placed on the couch in front of the parent.

5A. Which activity should the OTR encourage the infant to do as part of an intervention session for promoting the infant's oral motor skill development?

    A. Make funny faces in the mirror.

    B. Hum a simple song.

    C. Give kisses to a favorite toy.

    D. Suck a flavored ice pop.

Scenario B:

An OTR is completing an initial evaluation with a home health client who has stage 4 Parkinson's disease. The client walks with a festinating gait using the support of furniture and walls to maintain balance when walking from room to room. The house is cluttered, has poor lighting in hallways, and all rooms are carpeted except the bathroom. When asked about primary concerns, the client becomes tearful stating concerns about having frequent bladder accidents from not being able to get from the living room to the bathroom quickly enough. The client also reports difficulty changing the soiled clothing.

B1. Which strategy should the OTR recommend **INITIALLY** for reducing the frequency of the client's bladder accidents?

    A. Place a commode chair near the living room.

    B. Practice pelvic floor exercises on a daily basis.

    C. Reduce intake of fluids during the evening.

    D. Void every 2 hours throughout the day.

B2. Which clothing modification would be **MOST BENEFICIAL** for the OTR to recommend for enabling the client to successfully complete lower body dressing and undressing activities?

    A. Switch from wearing belted pants to wearing pants with an elastic waistband.

    B. Replace the zippers and buttons on the pants with hook and loop closures.

    C. Use a button hook to fasten the buttons on pant waistbands.

    D. Attach a zipper pull to the zipper tab on front-opening pants.

B3. Which environmental modification should the OTR recommend **INITIALLY** in order to maximize the client's mobility within the home?

    A. Replace carpet with anti-skid strips throughout the home.

    B. Clear pathways leading to routinely used rooms in the house.

    C. Install an ECU to operate lights, television and phone systems.

    D. Raise the height of bedroom and living room furniture.

B4. After a 2-week period a reevaluation reveals the client continues to have frequent bladder accidents. What action should the OTR take **NEXT** based on this information?

    A. Report the findings to the client's primary care physician.

    B. Discuss additional home modifications with a family member.

    C. Recommend a referral for the client to attend an adult day care facility.

    D. Suggest the client use an external catheter for bladder management.

B5. Which administrative task **MUST** the OTR complete in order to maximize reimbursement by Medicare for services provided to this client?

    A. Write a weekly summary of observed client changes between visits.

    B. Provide justification for maintenance activities that promote aging in place.

    C. Document each visit including client's response to skilled services provided.

    D. Update the plan of care whenever the client's functional level changes.

Scenario C:

A patient has hemiplegia secondary to a right CVA one week ago. The patient transferred from an acute care setting to an inpatient rehabilitation facility one day ago. Medical history indicates the patient has a pre-existing peripheral neuropathy and glaucoma. Prior to admission to the acute care hospital, the patient lived in a first-floor apartment and had just started using a standard wheelchair for community mobility due to unrelenting neuralgia. Discharge documentation from the acute care facility indicates the patient has moderate spasticity of the affected side, requires moderate assistance with transfers, dressing and bathing; and minimum assistance with grooming and self-feeding. During the initial interprofessional team meeting, the social worker indicates the patient wants to return home and the spouse will provide primary caregiving responsibilities. Additionally, the spouse asked if the patient can continue to use the standard wheelchair they already own for in-home and community outings.

C1. Which type of assessment would be **MOST BENEFICIAL** for the OTR to administer for acquiring information about and tracking the status of the patient's visual-perceptual abilities?

   A. Standardized ADL neurobehavioral evaluation
   B. Skilled observation during typical daily routines
   C. Functional independence measure
   D. Series of occupation-based screenings

C2. Which type of transfer surface is **BEST** to use when starting to teach the patient the sit-to-stand phase of a functional transfer?

   A. Bedside chair with a cushioned seat and back
   B. Edge of a hospital bed elevated to maximal height
   C. Standard sling-seat wheelchair with swing-out leg rests
   D. Mat table with high-low height adjustments

C3. Which transfer technique should the OTR teach the spouse to use when assisting the patient to transition from wheelchair to bed?

   A. Sliding board
   B. Stand-pivot
   C. Bent pivot
   D. Mechanical lift

NBCOT Study Guide - OTR Certification Examination   111   Scenario Samples

C4. Which of the following mobility devices would be **MOST BENEFICIAL** for the patient to learn to use in preparation for return to home?

    A. Standard wheelchair with wedge cushion and pneumatic tires

    B. Power mobility scooter with a rechargeable battery pack

    C. Wheelchair with solid-seat and removable armrests and footrests

    D. Power wheelchair with folding frame and a contoured seat

C5. What information should the OTR include in **INITIAL** documentation to meet Medicare reimbursement criteria?

    A. Report of functional outcomes using the Minimum Data Set (MDS) — Medicare & Medicad SNFs

    B. Results from portions of the Outcome and Assessment Information Set (OASIS) — Home Health

    C. Baseline measure of functional independence using a Patient Assessment Instrument (PAI)

    D. Expected intervention outcomes based on results from Resource Utilization Groups (RUGS) → SNFs

Scenario D:

A patient who has a complete T_{12} paraplegia has recently undergone a coronary artery bypass graft surgery following a myocardial infarction. The patient is referred to occupational therapy one day after surgery. Review of the medical record indicates the patient lives alone and was independent in all IADL prior to the myocardial infarction. The patient plans to resume work in a call center and enjoys competing in wheelchair races.

D1. Which of the following assessments is **CONTRAINDICATED** to include in an initial evaluation with this patient?

    A. Observation of BADL

    B. Manual muscle test

    C. Upper body ROM

    D. Semi structured interview

D2. The patient's heart rate increases by 15 beats per minute above resting heart rate when completing upper body dressing while seated in a wheelchair at bedside. Which action should the OTR take in response to this observation?

    A. Encourage the patient to complete the dressing activity.

    B. Stop the activity and assist the patient to return to bed.

    C. Seek medical assistance and monitor blood pressure.

    D. Elevate the patient's legs until heart rate returns to normal.

D3. Which intervention is **MOST BENEFICIAL** for the patient to learn during the initial stage of Phase I of cardiac rehabilitation?

    A. Upper body graded exercise and strengthening program

    B. Methods for monitoring responses during modified transfers

    C. Energy conservation techniques to use during functional activities

    D. Pursed lip breathing techniques for use during functional activities

D4. What information is **MOST IMPORTANT** for the OTR to provide during a pre-discharge interprofessional team meeting?

    A. Location of community-based cardiac rehabilitation programs in the area

    B. The patient's desire to resume training for an upcoming wheelchair race

    C. Modifications required at the call center prior to the patient's return to work

    D. Patient's cardiac tolerance during completion of basic self-care activities

D5. What information should the OTR include in a letter of justification to a third-party payer to increase the likelihood of reimbursement for the patient's durable medical equipment needs?

    A. Rate of recovery and progress of the patient during Phase I cardiac rehabilitation

    B. Durable medical equipment vendors that can deliver the bed to the patient's home

    C. Assistive technology the patient is currently using to complete self-care activities

    D. Purpose of the bed in enabling the patient to continue sternal precautions

Scenario E:

A young adult patient is in an acute rehabilitation facility after sustaining a focal brain injury as a result of a fall while playing football. Medical records indicate the injuries resulted in a subdural hematoma and the patient is currently functioning at Level VI (Confused-appropriate) on the Rancho Los Amigos scale. The discharge plan is for the patient to return home to live with both parents who will provide caregiver assistance.

E1. Which type of motor response is characteristic for this type of trauma?

    A. Loss of voluntary muscle control with associated hyperreflexia

    B. Cogwheel rigidity with associated hyporeflexia

    C. Decorticate rigidity with associated hyperreflexia

    D. Involuntary muscle control with accompanying hyporeflexia

E2. Which information would be **MOST BENEFICIAL** to use when prioritizing the patient's intervention goals and selecting activities as part of the initial intervention plan?

    A. Patient's level of insight regarding the influence of current condition on occupational roles

    B. Physical readiness and patient's motivation to begin a wheelchair mobility training program

    C. Influence of current neurobehavioral skills on functional task completion

    D. Parental report of the patient's pre-morbid cognitive skills and abilities

E3. Which activity provides the **MOST** information about the patient's current cognitive skills?

    A. Preparing a favorite cold snack and beverage

    B. Playing beginner-level football video games

    C. Text-messaging friends on a smart phone

    D. Catching and throwing a ball at a target

E4. Which type of activity would be **BEST** for the parents to use when visiting the patient at the facility during evenings and weekends?

    A. Age-appropriate board games with standard rules

    B. Simple card games requiring recognition and matching

    C. Computerized games that provide immediate feedback

    D. Watching a favorite team play football on television

E5. What information is **MOST IMPORTANT** for the OTR to provide to the parents during discharge planning?

- A. Post-acute rehabilitation and home program resources
- B. Methods for identifying and monitoring caregiving fatigue
- C. Patient's maximum future vocational potential
- D. Ongoing effects of patient's injury on family dynamics

Scenario F:

An OTR working in a home health setting is evaluating a client who has COPD. The client uses a pulse oximeter for self-monitoring and supplemental oxygen through nasal cannula as needed. The client lives alone in a single-level home, has meals delivered by a community outreach service and uses public transportation for community mobility. The client is independent with BADL but notes these tasks take longer due to fatigue and shortness of breath. The client's goal is to remain independent and to continue caring for a small pet dog.

F1. What information is **MOST IMPORTANT** for the OTR to include as part of the client instruction during the initial intervention sessions with this client?

- A. Procedures for accessing community resources to help with pet management
- B. Upper extremity strengthening exercises to complete for increasing endurance
- C. Adaptive equipment that would be beneficial to use during BADL and IADL
- D. Methods for managing energy expenditure during typical daily tasks

F2. During a meal preparation task, the client becomes short of breath and confused. What **INITIAL** action should the OTR take in response to this observation?

- A. Alert the client's home health nurse.
- B. Cue the client to modify breathing techniques.
- C. Ask the client to rate the level of dyspnea.
- D. Check the client's level of oxygenation.

F3. Which breathing technique should the OTR instruct the client to use to improve oxygenation?

- A. Breathe in through the nose and mouth; exhale through the nose.
- B. Breathe in slowly through the nose; exhale through pursed lips.
- C. Place hands on hips and extend the spine while breathing in and out.
- D. Elevate the diaphragm when inhaling; depress when exhaling.

F4. Which compensatory technique should the client learn to use during BADL tasks?

   A. Support the elbows on the sink to brush teeth with an electric toothbrush.

   B. Inhale slowly while reaching down to the feet to put on shoes and socks.

   C. Exhale while reaching for a pair of shoes from a high shelf in a closet.

   D. Use a button hook to button and unbutton front-opening shirts.

F5. Which technique would be **MOST BENEFICIAL** for the client to use when taking the dog for a walk?

   A. Autogenic training techniques

   B. Progressive muscle relaxation

   C. Diaphragmatic breathing

   D. Visualization techniques

Scenario G:

An adolescent sustained a non-displaced fracture of the radial head of the dominant arm one month ago. Initial treatment included long-arm casting for 2 weeks followed by half-cast splinting during activities. The adolescent was referred to OT due to a progressive increase in pain of the affected arm; despite evidence of fracture healing. During the initial evaluation, the OTR observes the adolescent holds the affected extremity in a protected position and prefers to use the non-dominant hand for functional tasks. Observation of the adolescent's ROM indicates full active ROM of the right shoulder, approximately -15° of elbow extension and 90° of elbow flexion. When the adolescent attempts to make a fist, composite finger flexion of the index through small finger measures one-inch (2.5 cm) from the fingertip to distal palmar crease. Wrist extension and flexion appear to be within functional limits; but the adolescent refuses to allow the OTR to complete goniometric measurements. The affected hand is warm to touch, with mottled skin and moderate pitting edema of the hand, fingers, and elbow. One of the adolescent's goals is to resume participation on the school gymnastics team.

G1. In addition to having decreased functional ROM secondary to the fracture, what is the adolescent's clinical presentation **MOST** consistent with?

    A. Atrophy resulting from disuse

    B. Chiralgia paresthetica — snuffbox area, hand cuffs.

    C. Complex regional pain syndrome

    D. Interstitial compartment syndrome — compression of extremities
      athletes

G2. Along with promoting engagement in purposeful activity, which intervention should be included as part of the **INITIAL** intervention for managing the adolescent's clinical symptoms?

    A. Contrast baths and progressive resistive exercises

    B. Protective splinting and passive ROM exercises

    C. Long-arm serial casting and thermal ultrasound

    D. Graded manual edema mobilization and active ROM

G3. What is the **MOST** accurate method for measuring change in edema in the adolescent's hand?

    A. Circumferential measurements of the hands

    B. Amount of water displacement in a volumeter

    C. Tracings of the hand positioned prone on paper

    D. Ruler measurement of composite finger flexion

G4. Which of the following activities would be **MOST BENEFICIAL** to include as part of the home program for promoting a change in the adolescent's sympathetic nervous system responses during the initial phase of intervention?

A. Drawing and erasing pictures on a large dry erase board while in quadruped on the floor

B. Carrying a 10-lb (4.5 kg) with the affected hand for 15-minute intervals several times a day

C. Throwing a light weight ball at a target placed at varying distances from the adolescent

D. Playing an interactive computer sports game with a friend or family member

G5. Which activity would support the gymnastics goal and would be effective to include as part of the intervention when the adolescent transitions to the **NEXT** stage of the diagnoses?

A. Walking across a 3-inch (7.6 cm) wide balance beam

B. Tumbling forward across a mat in the gym

C. Hanging and gently swinging from a parallel bar

D. Swinging both legs while straddling a pommel horse

Scenario H:

A resident in a long-term care facility has amyotrophic lateral sclerosis (ALS). Functional muscle strength of both upper extremities is Fair minus (3-/5) bilaterally. The resident currently uses both lower extremities to propel a standard manual wheelchair for short distances within the facility and requires moderate assistance of one person during functional transfers. The resident notes a recent increase of coughing when eating, difficulty holding built-up utensils at mealtime, and recurrent lower extremity muscle cramps and increased fatigue. These changes now interfere with the ability to navigate the current wheelchair to the dining room and to eat meals independently.

H1. Which of the following symptoms of this disease **TYPICALLY** impacts functional performance?

A. Neuralgia and blurred vision

B. Fasciculations and muscle atrophy

C. Intention tremor and bradykinesia

D. Peripheral neuropathy and hyporeflexia

H2. What is the **MOST** probable cause for this resident's coughing during meal times?

A. Decreased tongue control

B. Hyperactive gag reflex

C. Environmental distractions

D. Poor lip closure

H3. What is the **MOST IMPORTANT** safety recommendation for the resident to follow during meal times?

A. Sit fully upright and tuck chin when swallowing.

B. Eat warmed foods that have a pureed consistency.

C. Eat in a quiet environment away from distractions.

D. Use assistive devices to minimize muscle fatigue.

H4. What additional action should the OTR take to enable the resident to maintain independence during meals?

A. Provide a swivel spoon to use with pureed foods.

B. Teach compensatory strategies to support the proximal arms when eating.

C. Provide the resident with a mechanical feeder during meals.

D. Assess the need for a mobile arm support and universal cuff.

H5. What additional action should the OTR take **NEXT** based on the resident's current mobility status?

A. Order a customized contour insert for the current wheelchair.

B. Determine medical necessity for power mobility options.

C. Add a lap tray to the current wheelchair for increased postural support.

D. Arrange for a care provider to wheel the resident to meals.

SECTION 8

Answer Key for OTR Multiple-Choice Study Items in Scenario Format

Scenario: A	
#	Correct Answer
1.	D
2.	A
3.	D
4.	B
5.	C

Scenario: B	
#	Correct Answer
1.	D
2.	A
3.	B
4.	A
5.	C

Scenario: C	
#	Correct Answer
1.	A
2.	D
3.	B
4.	C
5.	C

Scenario: D	
#	Correct Answer
1.	B
2.	A
3.	B
4.	D
5.	D

Scenario: E	
#	Correct Answer
1.	A
2.	C
3.	A
4.	B
5.	A

Scenario: F	
#	Correct Answer
1.	D
2.	D
3.	B
4.	A
5.	C

Scenario: G	
#	Correct Answer
1.	C
2.	D
3.	B
4.	A
5.	C

Scenario: H	
#	Correct Answer
1.	B
2.	A
3.	A
4.	D
5.	B

OTR Scenario-Format Multiple-Choice Sample Items

Answers, Rationales, and References

SCENARIO A:

1A. Correct Answer: D

Postural alignment and trunk stability influence oral motor control and distal extremity control. It is important for the OTR to assess these prior to starting an oral-motor feeding program.

Domain: 01

Reference: Case-Smith, J., O'Brien, J. (2010). *Occupational Therapy for Children* (6th ed.). St. Louis, MO: Elsevier Mosby. Pages 454-455.

2A. Correct Answer: A

The early intervention process recognizes that parents can be the most effective facilitator of change. It is therefore important to ascertain the specific childrearing beliefs and family routines when collaborating with parents on designing an intervention plan for the infant.

Domain: 01

Reference: Case-Smith, J., O'Brien, J. (2010). *Occupational Therapy for Children* (6th ed.). St. Louis, MO: Elsevier Mosby. Page 457.

3A. Correct Answer: D

Encouraging the infant to explore the mouth using a rubber toy dipped in applesauce is an effective way to desensitize and build up the infant's tolerance to oral feeding.

Domain: 03

Reference: Case-Smith, J., O'Brien, J. (2010). *Occupational Therapy for Children* (6th ed.). St. Louis, MO: Elsevier Mosby. Pages 460-461.

4A. Correct Answer: B

Placing the infant in a car seat during feeding activities is the best method to achieve postural stability and alignment for feeding.

Domain: 03

Reference: Case-Smith, J., O'Brien, J. (2010). *Occupational Therapy for Children* (6th ed.). St. Louis, MO: Elsevier Mosby. Pages 458-459.

5A. Correct Answer: C

Kissing is an activity that encourages active lip movements and can be used to supplement other oral motor developmental activities.

Domain: 03

Reference: Case-Smith, J., O'Brien, J. (2010). *Occupational Therapy for Children* (6th ed.). St. Louis, MO: Elsevier Mosby. Page 469.

B1. Correct Answer: D

A scheduled voiding program will help to minimize overfilling of the bladder and reduce the incidence of bladder accidents. The client will not be in a rush to walk to the bathroom if the bladder is not overfull.

Domain: 03

Reference: Pendleton, H.M., Schultz-Krohn, W. (eds). (2013). *Pedretti's Occupational Therapy: Practice Skills for Physical Dysfunction* (7th ed.). St. Louis, MO: Elsevier Mosby. Page 852.

Smith-Gabai, H. (2011). *Occupational Therapy in Acute Care*. Bethesda, MD: AOTA Press. Page 598.

B2. Correct Answer: A

One of the symptoms of stage 4 Parkinson's disease is severely compromised fine motor skills. Wearing pants with an elastic waistband will help the client to complete lower body dressing without relying on fine motor skills to fasten regular or adapted closures.

Domain: 03

Reference: Pendleton, H.M., Schultz-Krohn, W. (eds). (2013). *Pedretti's Occupational Therapy: Practice Skills for Physical Dysfunction* (7th ed.). St. Louis, MO: Elsevier Mosby. Pages 942-944, 204.

B3. Correct Answer: B

Due to the client's festinating gait, the client is at a greater risk for falls. Clearing pathways in the house should be done **INITIALLY** to help to reduce the client's risk of falls. An ECU may be a helpful device for the client and can be considered after ensuring commonly used pathways in the home are cleared.

Domain: 03

Reference: Pendleton, H.M., Schultz-Krohn, W. (eds). (2013). *Pedretti's Occupational Therapy: Practice Skills for Physical Dysfunction* (7th ed.). St. Louis, MO: Elsevier Mosby. Pages 50, 942-944, 239.

B4. Correct Answer: A

The OTR should report the reevaluation results to the client's primary care physician. Changes in the autonomic nervous system – including bladder function – are common with the progression of Parkinson's disease and may require medication management.

Domain: 02

Reference: Smith-Gabai, H. (2011). *Occupational Therapy in Acute Care*. Bethesda, MD: AOTA Press. Pages 397, 399, 404.

B5. Correct Answer: C

In the home health setting, a separate note must document each visit. This should include medically necessary skilled services provided and the client's response to these services.

Domain: 04

Reference: Pendleton, H.M., Schultz-Krohn, W. (eds). (2013). *Pedretti's Occupational Therapy: Practice Skills for Physical Dysfunction* (7th ed.). St. Louis, MO: Elsevier Mosby. Page 129.

SCENARIO C:

C1. Correct Answer: A

Visual perceptual skills involve the processing of visual information by the brain and motor response. Using a standardized ADL assessment would provide the most objective information about the patient's current visual-perceptual status. Results of this type of assessment can also used as a baseline for tracking changes in the patient's functional skills.

Domain: 01

Reference: Pendleton, H.M., Schultz-Krohn, W. (eds). (2013). *Pedretti's Occupational Therapy: Practice Skills for Physical Dysfunction* (7th ed.). St. Louis, MO: Elsevier Mosby. Page 633.

C2. Correct Answer: D

A high-low mat table provides a firm and stable surface from which to complete a transfer as well as enabling the OTR to grade the height of the surface to promote success with this task.

Domain: 03

Reference: Gillen, G. (2011). *Stroke Rehabilitation: A Function-Based Approach* (3rd ed.). St. Louis, MO: Elsevier Mosby. Pages 370-375.

C3. Correct Answer: B

This is the best transfer to teach the patient's spouse, as it enables the spouse to safely provide cueing and assistance to the patient during the transfer if needed.

Domain: 03

Reference: Gillen, G. (2011). *Stroke Rehabilitation: A Function-Based Approach* (3rd ed.). St. Louis, MO: Elsevier Mosby. Pages 370-375.

C4. Correct Answer: C

A wheelchair with a solid-seat insert promotes postural alignment. Removable armrests and footrests promote safety during functional transfers.

Domain: 03

Reference: Pendleton, H.M., Schultz-Krohn, W. (eds). (2013). *Pedretti's Occupational Therapy: Practice Skills for Physical Dysfunction* (7th ed.). St. Louis, MO: Elsevier Mosby. Pages 242-253.

C5. Correct Answer: C

Criteria for Medicare reimbursement for services provided at inpatient rehabilitation facilities is based – in part – on the measure of functional independence noted in the standard Patient Assessment Instrument (PAI).

Domain: 04

Reference: Gateley, C., Borcherding, S. (2012). *Documentation Manual for Occupational Therapy: Writing SOAP Notes* (3rd ed.). Thorofare, NJ: SLACK, Inc. Pages 13-14.

SCENARIO D:

D1. Correct Answer: B

Manual muscle testing requires exertion of maximal effort to determine accurate strength levels. Although patients are instructed to exhale during testing, it is not uncommon for patients to hold their breath while exerting effort during the test. Holding the breath or sustaining an isometric contraction is contraindicated for patients who have recently undergone cardiac surgery. Additionally, one-sided pulling or pushing actions with the arms must be avoided for up to 6 weeks following surgery.

Domain: 01

Reference: Smith-Gabai, H. (2011). *Occupational Therapy in Acute Care*. Bethesda, MD: AOTA Press. Pages 118-119.

D2. Correct Answer: A

This is a normal response to this level of activity. When completing activities during the first 2 weeks of recovery after cardiac surgery, the heart rate should not increase more than 30 beats per minute above resting rate.

Domain: 01

Reference: Smith-Gabai, H. (2011). *Occupational Therapy in Acute Care*. Bethesda, MD: AOTA Press. Pages 118-119.

D3. Correct Answer: B

The primary focus during phase I cardiac rehabilitation is to provide the patient with guidelines for monitoring response to low level activity; including self-care and transfers.

Domain: 03

Reference: Pendleton, H.M., Schultz-Krohn, W. (eds). (2013). *Pedretti's Occupational Therapy: Practice Skills for Physical Dysfunction* (7th ed.). St. Louis, MO: Elsevier Mosby. Pages 1202-1204.

D4. Correct Answer: D

It is **MOST IMPORTANT** for the OTR to report the patient's cardiac tolerance during BADL. This provides the team with guidance about the amount of caregiving and/or family support the patient will need at the time of discharge.

Domain: 02

Reference: Pendleton, H.M., Schultz-Krohn, W. (eds). (2013). *Pedretti's Occupational Therapy: Practice Skills for Physical Dysfunction* (7th ed.). St. Louis, MO: Elsevier Mosby. Page 1210.

D5. Correct Answer: D

A letter of justification to third-party payers should include a statement of medical necessity related to the patient's functional skills and abilities.

Domain: 04

Reference: Gateley, C., Borcherding, S. (2012). *Documentation Manual for Occupational Therapy: Writing SOAP Notes* (3rd ed.). Thorofare, NJ: SLACK, Inc. Pages 9, 55.

SCENARIO E:

E1. Correct Answer: A

This type of brain injury is typically characterized by a loss of voluntary muscle control and hyperreflexia due to upper motor neuron involvement.

Domain: 01

Reference: Pendleton, H.M., Schultz-Krohn, W. (eds). (2013). *Pedretti's Occupational Therapy: Practice Skills for Physical Dysfunction* (7th ed.). St. Louis, MO: Elsevier Mosby. Pages 884-891.

E2. Correct Answer: C

Having a clear understanding of the patient's neurobehavioral skills will allow the OTR to prioritize and structure intervention based on the patient's current needs and activity demands.

Domain: 02

Reference: Pendleton, H.M., Schultz-Krohn, W. (eds). (2013). *Pedretti's Occupational Therapy: Practice Skills for Physical Dysfunction* (7th ed.). St. Louis, MO: Elsevier Mosby. Pages 902-905.

E3. Correct Answer: A

The OTR can obtain valuable information about the patient's current cognitive skills by assessing the patient complete a simple ADL task. Using this task enables the OTR to assess the client's ability to sequence, follow instructions, attend to a specific task, and display appropriate safety and judgment.

Domain: 01

Reference: Pendleton, H.M., Schultz-Krohn, W. (eds). (2013). *Pedretti's Occupational Therapy: Practice Skills for Physical Dysfunction* (7th ed.). St. Louis, MO: Elsevier Mosby. Pages 902-905.

E4. Correct Answer: B

Card games are frequently used in the early stages of rehabilitation as they can be easily graded to the patient's current cognitive abilities. Card games are typical family occupations and enable the parents to actively engage in the patient's cognitive remediation.

Domain: 03

Reference: Pendleton, H.M., Schultz-Krohn, W. (eds). (2013). *Pedretti's Occupational Therapy: Practice Skills for Physical Dysfunction* (7th ed.). St. Louis, MO: Elsevier Mosby. Pages 902-905, 908-909.

E5. Correct Answer: A

The OTR should facilitate transition from the acute setting to the next level of care. It is important to educate the family about transitional resources for supporting the patient's continued progress.

Domain: 02

Reference: Pendleton, H.M., Schultz-Krohn, W. (eds). (2013). *Pedretti's Occupational Therapy: Practice Skills for Physical Dysfunction* (7th ed.). St. Louis, MO: Elsevier Mosby. Pages 911-912.

SCENARIO F:

F1. Correct Answer: D

It is **MOST IMPORTANT** for the client to learn to manage energy expenditure at this stage of the disease process. This information will help the client to perform at a higher functional level. The OTR can then introduce other interventions as needed.

Domain: 02

Reference: Pendleton, H.M., Schultz-Krohn, W. (eds). (2013). *Pedretti's Occupational Therapy: Practice Skills for Physical Dysfunction* (7th ed.). St. Louis, MO: Elsevier Mosby. Pages 1207, 1209-1210.

Smith-Gabai, H. (2011). *Occupational Therapy in Acute Care*. Bethesda, MD: AOTA Press. Pages 173-175.

F2. Correct Answer: D

Shortness of breath and confusion are signs of hypoxia. The OTR should check the client's oxygen saturation level to determine what further action should be taken.

Domain: 01

Reference: Pendleton, H.M., Schultz-Krohn, W. (eds). (2013). *Pedretti's Occupational Therapy: Practice Skills for Physical Dysfunction* (7th ed.). St. Louis, MO: Elsevier Mosby. Pages 1209-1210.

Smith-Gabai, H. (2011). *Occupational Therapy in Acute Care*. Bethesda, MD: AOTA Press. Pages 173-175.

F3. Correct Answer: B

To initiate pursed lip breathing, the client should inhale air slowly through the nose and exhale through the lips as though whistling. This technique increases breathing control and efficiency.

Domain: 03

Reference: Pendleton, H.M., Schultz-Krohn, W. (eds). (2013). *Pedretti's Occupational Therapy: Practice Skills for Physical Dysfunction* (7th ed.). St. Louis, MO: Elsevier Mosby. Pages 1209-1210.

Smith-Gabai, H. (2011). *Occupational Therapy in Acute Care.* Bethesda, MD: AOTA Press. Pages 173-175.

F4. Correct Answer: A

This is an energy conservation technique the client should use during BADL.

Domain: 03

Reference: Pendleton, H.M., Schultz-Krohn, W. (eds). (2013). *Pedretti's Occupational Therapy: Practice Skills for Physical Dysfunction* (7th ed.). St. Louis, MO: Elsevier Mosby. Pages 1209-1210.

Smith-Gabai, H. (2011). *Occupational Therapy in Acute Care.* Bethesda, MD: AOTA Press. Pages 173-175.

F5. Correct Answer: C

Diaphragmatic breathing is the **MOST BENEFICIAL** method for the client to use for controlling dyspnea during this daily task.

Domain: 03

Reference: Pendleton, H.M., Schultz-Krohn, W. (eds). (2013). *Pedretti's Occupational Therapy: Practice Skills for Physical Dysfunction* (7th ed.). St. Louis, MO: Elsevier Mosby. Pages 1209-1210.

Smith-Gabai, H. (2011). *Occupational Therapy in Acute Care.* Bethesda, MD: AOTA Press. Pages 173-175.

SCENARIO G:

G1. Correct Answer: C

Stage I complex regional pain syndrome is characterized by abnormal vasomotor and sudomotor activity, and pain that is disproportionate to the injury.

Domain: 02

Reference: Pendleton, H.M., Schultz-Krohn, W. (eds). (2013). *Pedretti's Occupational Therapy: Practice Skills for Physical Dysfunction* (7th ed.). St. Louis, MO: Elsevier Mosby. Pages 1062-1063.

G2. Correct Answer: D

Graded manual edema mobilization (MEM) and active ROM will help to interrupt the pain cycle during this phase of CRPS. Graded MEM techniques and ROM should be used based on the adolescent's ability to tolerate touch and movement.

Domain: 02

Reference: Pendleton, H.M., Schultz-Krohn, W. (eds). (2013). *Pedretti's Occupational Therapy: Practice Skills for Physical Dysfunction* (7th ed.). St. Louis, MO: Elsevier Mosby. Pages 1062-1063.

G3. Correct Answer: B

Volumetric measurements and circumferential measurements are typically used to measure edema. Of these measurement techniques, volumetric measurements are more accurate.

Domain: 01

Reference: Pendleton, H.M., Schultz-Krohn, W. (eds). (2013). *Pedretti's Occupational Therapy: Practice Skills for Physical Dysfunction* (7th ed.). St. Louis, MO: Elsevier Mosby. Pages 1046-1047.

G4. Correct Answer: A

Stress-loading and scrubbing-type exercises should be initiated during this stage of the adolescent's rehabilitation. Analyzing the activities listed, option A represents a scrubbing-type exercise that can be easily graded based on the adolescent's current pain symptoms. Although option B represents a stress-loading exercise, the weight is too heavy for this stage of the adolescent's rehabilitation.

Domain: 01

Reference: Pendleton, H.M., Schultz-Krohn, W. (eds). (2013). *Pedretti's Occupational Therapy: Practice Skills for Physical Dysfunction* (7th ed.). St. Louis, MO: Elsevier Mosby. Pages 1046-1047.

G5. Correct Answer: C

Traction can be used in addition to a stress-loading program to promote positive sympathetic nervous system changes. In a supervised context, hanging and swinging form a parallel bar will provide this input, assist with increasing ROM and functional grip, and progress the adolescent toward the goal of resuming gymnastics.

Domain: 01

Reference: Pendleton, H.M., Schultz-Krohn, W. (eds). (2013). *Pedretti's Occupational Therapy: Practice Skills for Physical Dysfunction* (7th ed.). St. Louis, MO: Elsevier Mosby. Pages 1046-1047.

SCENARIO H:

H1. Correct Answer: B

Fasciculations and muscle atrophy are characteristic symptoms of ALS. Sensation, vision, and bowel and bladder control are typically not affected.

Domain: 01

Reference: Pendleton, H.M., Schultz-Krohn, W. (eds). (2013). *Pedretti's Occupational Therapy: Practice Skills for Physical Dysfunction* (7th ed.). St. Louis, MO: Elsevier Mosby. Pages 919-920.

H2. Correct Answer: A

The tongue moves the food in the mouth in preparation for swallowing. In ALS, weakness of the oral musculature can result in an inability of the person to adequately move food in the mouth in preparation for swallowing.

Domain: 03

Reference: Pendleton, H.M., Schultz-Krohn, W. (eds). (2013). *Pedretti's Occupational Therapy: Practice Skills for Physical Dysfunction* (7th ed.). St. Louis, MO: Elsevier Mosby. Pages 919-920.

H3. Correct Answer: A

Head and neck positioning have a direct effect on the patient's ability to swallow and manage secretions. Incorrect positioning can lead to coughing and aspiration.

Domain: 03

Reference: Pendleton, H.M., Schultz-Krohn, W. (eds). (2013). *Pedretti's Occupational Therapy: Practice Skills for Physical Dysfunction* (7th ed.). St. Louis, MO: Elsevier Mosby. Pages 698-699, 919-921.

H4. Correct Answer: D

A mobile arm support and a universal cuff are indicated based on the resident's current functional muscle strength and difficulty using current adaptive eating utensils.

Domain: 04

Reference: Radomski, M., Trombly-Latham, C. (2008). *Occupational Therapy for Physical Dysfunction* (6th ed.). Baltimore, MD: Wolters Kluwer, Lippincott, Williams & Wilkins. Pages 200, 783-793.

H5. Correct Answer: B

Considering the resident's functional decline and the progressive nature of ALS, the OTR should determine the medical necessity for power mobility to enable independence with basic mobility, improve respiratory function for preventing aspiration, and maintain skin integrity.

Domain: 03

Reference: Pendleton, H.M., Schultz-Krohn, W. (eds). (2013). *Pedretti's Occupational Therapy: Practice Skills for Physical Dysfunction* (7th ed.).St. Louis, MO: Elsevier Mosby. Pages 243-244.

Radomski, M., Trombly-Latham, C. (2008). *Occupational Therapy for Physical Dysfunction* (6th ed.). Baltimore, MD: Wolters Kluwer, Lippincott, Williams & Wilkins. Pages 492-493.

APPENDIX A

2012 Validated Domain, Task, and Knowledge Statements for the OTR

2012 Validated Domain, Task and Knowledge Statements for the OTR

Domains are specified in bold with a two-digit number, tasks are grouped under each domain (four-digit number), and the tasks' associated knowledge and skill statements are listed with a six-digit number.

Code	Description
	DOMAIN 1
01	**Acquire information regarding factors that influence occupational performance throughout the occupational therapy process.**
0101	**Acquire information about a client's functional skills, roles, context, and prioritized needs through the use of available resources and standardized and non-standardized assessments in order to develop an occupational profile.**
010101	Normal development and function across the lifespan
010102	Expected patterns, progressions, and prognoses associated with conditions that limit occupational performance (e.g., stages of disease, secondary complications, outcomes)
010103	Processes and procedures for acquiring client information (e.g., client records, observation, interview, occupational profile)
010104	Administration, scoring, purpose, indications, advantages, and limitations of standardized and non-standardized screening and assessment tools
010105	Influence of client factors, context, and environment on habits, routines, roles, and rituals
010106	Methods for recognizing and responding to typical and atypical physiological, cognitive, and behavioral conditions
0102	**Analyze evidence obtained from the occupational profile to identify factors that influence a client's occupational performance.**
010201	Therapeutic application of theoretical approaches, models of practice, and frames of reference
010202	Activity analysis in relation to the occupational profile, practice setting, and stage of occupational therapy process
010203	Internal and external influences on occupational performance (e.g., environment, context, condition, medication, other therapies)
	DOMAIN 2
02	**Formulate conclusions regarding client needs and priorities to develop and monitor an intervention plan throughout the occupational therapy process.**
0201	**Analyze and interpret standardized and non-standardized assessment results, using information obtained about the client's current condition, context, and priorities in order to develop and manage client-centered intervention plans.**
020101	Methods for analyzing results from screening and assessments

Code	Description
020102	Integration of screening and assessment results with client occupational profile, client condition, expected outcomes, and level of service delivery to develop a targeted action plan, monitor progress, and reassess the plan
020103	Methods for determining program development and client advocacy needs (e.g., aging in place, falls prevention, health and wellness programs, community support groups, inservices)
0202	**Collaborate with the client, the client's relevant others, occupational therapy colleagues, and other professionals and staff, using a client-centered approach to manage occupational therapy services guided by evidence and principles of best practice.**
020201	Interprofessional roles, responsibilities, and care coordination (e.g., referral to and consultation with other services)
020202	Management of collaborative client-centered intervention and transition plans based on client skills, abilities, and expected outcomes in relation to level of service delivery, frequency and duration of intervention, and available resources (includes communication with family, caregiver, and relevant others)
020203	Prioritization of goals based on client skills, abilities, and expected outcomes in relation to level of service delivery and frequency and duration of intervention (e.g., expected length of stay, transition plan)
	DOMAIN 3
03	**Select interventions for managing a client-centered plan throughout the occupational therapy process.**
0301	**Manage interventions for the infant, child, or adolescent client, using clinical reasoning, the intervention plan, and best practice standards consistent with pediatric condition(s) and typical developmental milestones (e.g., motor, sensory, psychosocial, and cognitive) in order to support participation within areas of occupation.**
030101	Influence of pediatric condition(s) and typical developmental milestones on areas of occupation
030102	Intervention activities for supporting participation in occupations based on current sensory, cognitive, motor, and psychosocial skills and abilities
030103	Intervention methods for facilitating or inhibiting sensory, motor, or perceptual processing based on pediatric condition(s), tasks, and environmental demands
030104	Intervention methods for improving range of motion, strength, and activity tolerance based on pediatric condition(s) in order to promote occupational performance
030105	Group facilitation methods appropriate to pediatric condition(s) and developmental level

Code	Description
030106	Splint design and fabrication, and types, functions, and use of orthotic and prosthetic devices based on pediatric condition(s) and task demands
030107	Assistive technology, adaptive devices, and durable medical equipment based on pediatric condition(s), task, and environmental demands
030108	Methods for adapting intervention techniques, activities, and environments in response to behaviors and developmental needs
030109	Intervention methods for enabling feeding and eating skills based on pediatric condition(s) and developmental level
030110	Transfer and positioning techniques based on pediatric condition(s), task, and environmental demands
030111	Prevocational and vocational interventions that support transition planning
030112	Seating options, positioning devices, and mobility systems based on pediatric condition(s), developmental level, and environmental demands
030113	Environmental modifications for maximizing accessibility and mobility within various contexts based on pediatric condition(s), developmental level, and task demands
030114	Methods for adapting or grading an activity, task, or an environment based on pediatric condition(s), developmental needs, and task demands
030115	Methods and techniques for promoting the continuation of the interventions within multiple contexts based on current pediatric condition(s), developmental level, and expected outcomes (e.g., home program, caregiver instructions, teacher consultation)
0302	**Manage interventions for the young, middle-aged, or older adult client, using clinical reasoning, the intervention plan, and best practice standards consistent with general medical, neurological, and musculoskeletal condition(s) in order to achieve functional outcomes within areas of occupation.**
030201	Influence of medical, neurological, and musculoskeletal condition(s) on activity selection and areas of occupation
030202	Rehabilitative strategies and procedures specific to medical, neurological, and musculoskeletal condition(s) (e.g., joint protection, work simplification, energy conservation)
030203	Methods and strategies for improving range of motion, strength, and activity tolerance based on general medical, neurological, and musculoskeletal condition(s) in order to promote occupational performance
030204	Strategies and procedures for facilitating or inhibiting sensory, motor, and perceptual processing based on general medical, neurological, and musculoskeletal condition(s)

Code	Description
030205	Methods for selecting and effectively applying superficial and deep thermal, mechanical, and electrotherapeutic physical agent modalities as an adjunct to participation in an activity
030206	Splint design and fabrication, and types, functions, and use of orthotic and prosthetic devices based on general medical, neurological, and musculoskeletal condition(s) and task demands
030207	Assistive technology (i.e., high and low tech), adaptive devices, and durable medical equipment based on client needs and general medical, neurological, and musculoskeletal condition(s)
030208	Intervention methods for enabling feeding and eating skills based on client needs and medical, neurological, and musculoskeletal condition(s)
030209	Transfer methods and positioning techniques based on client needs; general medical, neurological, and musculoskeletal condition(s); task; and environmental demands
030210	Seating options, positioning devices, and mobility systems based on client needs; medical, neurological, and musculoskeletal condition(s); task; and environmental demands
030211	Environmental modifications for maximizing accessibility and mobility within context based on client needs; medical, neurological, and musculoskeletal condition(s); and task demands
030212	Ergonomic principles and universal design for health promotion and injury prevention
030213	Methods for adapting and grading tasks and activities based on client needs and medical, neurological, and musculoskeletal condition(s)
030214	Methods and strategies for promoting the continuation of the intervention within context based on medical condition(s) and expected outcomes (e.g., home program, caregiver instructions)
0303	**Manage interventions for the young, middle-aged, and older adult client, using clinical reasoning, the intervention plan, and best practice standards consistent with psychosocial, cognitive, and developmental abilities in order to achieve functional outcomes within areas of occupation.**
030301	Influence of psychosocial, cognitive, and developmental abilities on areas of occupation
030302	Methods for facilitating groups to enhance participants' psychosocial, cognitive, and developmental skills
030303	Approaches (e.g., remediation, compensation, prevention) and interventions (e.g., problem solving, medication management, memory strategies) appropriate for psychosocial and cognitive models of practice (e.g., cognitive, behavioral, acquisitional, developmental)

Code	Description
030304	Environmental modifications to enhance community safety and well-being consistent with occupational roles and client needs
030305	Assistive technology and adaptive devices to enhance participation in occupation consistent with psychosocial, cognitive, and developmental abilities
030306	Methods for adapting and grading an intervention based on psychosocial, cognitive, and developmental abilities
030307	Methods and techniques for promoting the continuation of the interventions within multiple contexts based on psychosocial, cognitive, and developmental abilities (e.g., home program, caregiver instructions, job coach)

	DOMAIN 4
04	**Manage and direct occupational therapy services to promote quality in practice.**
0401	**Maintain and enhance competence, using professional development activities relevant to practice, job responsibilities, and regulatory body in order to provide evidence-based services.**
040101	Professional development activities
040102	Methods of analyzing and interpreting research and its application to practice
040103	Methods for evaluating, monitoring, and documenting service competency (e.g., self-assessment, peer review)
0402	**Manage occupational therapy service provision in accordance with laws, regulations, accreditation guidelines, and facility policies and procedures governing safe and ethical practice in order to protect consumers.**
040201	Influence of policies, procedures, and guidelines on service delivery
040202	Licensure laws, federally mandated requirements, and reimbursement policies related to occupational therapy service delivery (e.g., client confidentiality, levels of supervision, plan of care certification/recertification, referral policy)
040203	Methods for incorporating risk management techniques and monitoring safety related to occupational therapy service delivery
040204	Methods for applying continuous quality improvement processes and procedures to occupational therapy service delivery (e.g., program evaluation, outcome measures)
040205	Scope of practice and practice standards for occupational therapy (e.g., delegation, supervision, role delineation)
040206	Accountability processes and procedures using relevant technology (e.g., documentation guidelines, components of an intervention plan, coding systems, electronic medical records, written documentation)

APPENDIX B:

References

ACOTE. (2011). *Accreditation Standards for a Master's Degree Level Educational Program for the Occupational Therapist.* American Occupational Therapy Program.

Asher IE. (2007). *Occupational Therapy Assessment Tool: An Annotated Index* (3rd ed.). Bethesda, MD: AOTA Press.

*Barnhart PA. (1997). *The Guide to National Professional Certification Programs* (2nd ed.). Amherst, MA: HRD Press.

*Brookfield S. (1987). *Developing Critical Thinkers.* San Francisco, CA: Jossey-Bass, Inc.

Bonder BR. (2010). *Psychopathology and Function* (4th ed.). Thorofare, NJ: SLACK Inc.

Boyt-Schell B, Gillen G, Scaffa M, Cohn E. (2014). *Willard and Spackman's Occupational Therapy* (12th ed). Philadelphia, PA: Lippincott Williams &Wilkins.

Brown C, Stoffel V. (2011). *Occupational Therapy in Mental Health: A Vision for Participation.* Philadelphia: FA Davis.

Burke S, Higgins J, McClinton M, Saunders R, Valdata, L. (2006). *Hand and Upper Extremity Rehabilitation: A Practical Guide* (3rd ed.). St. Louis, MO: Elsevier, Churchill, Livingstone.

Cara E, MacRae A. (2013). *Psychosocial Occupational Therapy: An Evolving Practice* (3rd ed.). NY: Thomson Delmar.

Case-Smith J, O'Brien J. (2010). *Occupational Therapy for Children* (6th ed.). St. Louis, MO: Elsevier Mosby.

Cooper C. (2007). *Fundamentals of Hand Therapy: Clinical Reasoning and Treatment Guidelines for Common Diagnoses of the Upper Extremity.* St. Louis, MO: Elsevier Mosby.

Coppard BM, Lohman H. (2008). *Introduction to Splinting: A Clinical-Reasoning & Problem Solving Approach* (3rd ed.). St. Louis, MO: Elsevier Mosby.

*Covey SR. (1989). *The 7 Habits of Highly Effective People.* New York: Simon & Schuster.

Fazio L. (2008). *Developing Occupation-Centered Programming for the Community: A Workbook for Students and Professionals* (2nd ed.). Upper Saddle River, NJ: Prentice Hall.

Gateley C, Borcherding S. (2012). *Documentation Manual for Occupational Therapy* (3rd ed.). Thorofare, NJ: SLACK Inc.

Gillen G. (2011). *Stroke Rehabilitation: A Function-Based Approach* (3rd ed.). St. Louis, MO: Elsevier Mosby.

Kielhofner G. (2006). *Research in Occupational Therapy: Methods of Inquiry for Enhancing Practice*. Philadelphia: FA Davis.

*McClain N. Richardson B. & Wyatt J. (2004, May-June). *A profile of certification for pediatric nurses*. *Pediatric Nursing*, 207-211.

*Microsoft (2003). Microsoft certifications benefits of certification. Retrieved from www.microsoft.com/traincert.

NBCOT, Inc. (2013). *2013 Certification Renewal Handbook*. Gaithersburg, MD: NBCOT 2013 Publications.

Pendleton HM, Schultz-Krohn W (eds). (2013). *Pedretti's Occupational Therapy: Practice Skills for Physical Dysfunction* (7th ed.). St. Louis, MO: Elsevier Mosby.

Radomski MV, Trombly-Latham C. (2008). *Occupational Therapy for Physical Dysfunction* (6th ed.) Baltimore, MD: Wolters Kluwer, Lippincott, Williams &Wilkins.

Scaffa M, Reitz SM, Pizzi M. (2010). *Occupational Therapy in the Promotion of Health and Wellness*. Philadelphia, PA: FA Davis.

Sladyk K, Jacobs K, MacRae N. (2010). *Occupational Therapy Essentials for Clinical Competence*. Thorofare, NJ: SLACK Inc.

Smith-Gabai H. (2011). *Occupational Therapy in Acute Care*. Bethesda, MD: AOTA Press.

Zoltan B. (2007). *Vision, Perception, and Cognition: A Manual for the Evaluation and Treatment of the Adult with Acquired Brain Injury* (4th ed.). Thorofare, NJ: SLACK, Inc.

*References cited during introductory chapter of this study guide. These references should not be viewed as examination item references.

APPENDIX C:

Abbreviations and Acronyms

The following is a list of abbreviations and acronyms that may be used in examination items. Please note: The list provided in this Appendix is intended for study purposes only and is not comprehensive.

Abbreviation or Acronym	Expansion
ADA	The Americans with Disabilities Act
ADL	Activities of daily living
AIDS	Acquired immunodeficiency syndrome
ALS	Amyotrophic lateral sclerosis
BADL	Basic activities of daily living
COPD	Chronic obstructive pulmonary disease
COTA	CERTIFIED OCCUPATIONAL THERAPY ASSISTANT COTA®
CPR	Cardiopulmonary resuscitation
CRPS	Complex regional pain syndrome
CVA	Cerebrovascular accident
DIP	Distal interphalangeal*
DSM 5	Diagnostic and Statistical Manual of Mental Disorders - 5th Edition
HIPAA	Health Insurance Portability and Accountability Act
HIV	Human immunodeficiency virus
IADL	Instrumental activities of daily living
IDEA	Individuals with Disabilities Education Act
IEP	Individualized Education Program
MCP	Metacarpophalangeal*
OTR	OCCUPATIONAL THERAPIST REGISTERED OTR®
PIP	Proximal interphalangeal*
ROM	Range of motion
SCI	Spinal cord injury
SOAP	Subjective, Objective, Assessment, Plan (components of the problem-oriented medical record)

*Must be followed by the word "joint"

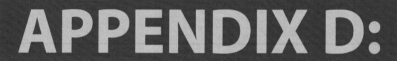

APPENDIX D:

Listing of common:

Diagnoses/Conditions

Intervention Applications/Equipment

Service Delivery Components

Roles and Responsibilities

Practice Settings/Situations

The following is a list of diagnoses / condition, intervention applications / equipment, service delivery components and setting that may be used as part of a multiple-choice examination item or clinical simulation problem. Please note: The lists provided in this Appendix are intended for study purposes only and are not comprehensive.

Diagnoses / Conditions

- Attention deficit hyperactivity disorder (ADHD)
- Acquired immunodeficiency syndrome (AIDS)
- Adjustment disorders
- Alcohol / substance abuse
- Alzheimer's disease
- Amyotrophic lateral sclerosis (ALS)
- Amputations (upper and lower extremity)
- Anxiety disorders
- Aphasia
- Apraxia (ideomotor / ideational)
- Arthritis (osteoarthritis / rheumatoid arthritis)
- Ataxia
- Autonomic dysreflexia
- Back pain
- Bipolar disorder
- Burns
- Cardiac / Cardiopulmonary disease
- Cerebral palsy
- Cerebrovascular Accident (CVA)
- Chronic Obstructive Pulmonary Disease (COPD)
- Cognitive dysfunction
- Complex regional pain syndrome (CRPS)
- Cumulative trauma disorders
    - deQuervain's tenosynovitis
    - Carpal tunnel syndrome
    - Lateral epicondylitis
    - Cubital tunnel syndrome
- Death and dying
- Decubitis ulcers
- Deep vein thrombosis
- Dementia / Alzheimer's disease / memory loss
- Depression
- Development (normal / abnormal)
- Developmental disorders
    - Autism spectrum disorder
    - Developmental delay
    - Down syndrome
- Diabetes
- Domestic violence / Abuse (child / spousal / elder)
- Dysphagia
- Dyspraxia
- Eating disorders
    - Anorexia
    - Bulemia
    - Obesity
- Edema
- Encephalopathy
- Failure to thrive

- Fall risk
- Fetal alcohol syndrome
- Fibromyalgia
- Fractures (upper and lower extremity)
- Guillain-Barré syndrome
- Hand injury
- Hemiplegia / hemiparesis
- Heterotropic ossification
- Human Immunodeficiency Virus (HIV)
- Hypertension / hypotension
- Hypertonia / spasticity
- Hypotonicity / flaccidity
- Intellectual disability
- Ischemia
- Joint replacement (hip / knee)
- Joints (MCP /PIP / DIP)
- Learning disabilities
- Low vision
- Muscular dystrophy
- Medication management (side effects)
- Multiple sclerosis
- Myasthenia gravis
- Nerve injuries / peripheral neuropathy
    - Median
    - Radial
    - Ulnar
- Normal child development
- Obsessive compulsive disorder (OCD)
- Oral motor dysfunction
- Osteoporosis
- Pain management
- Paralysis
- Parkinson's disease
- Perceptual disorders
- Perseveration
- Personality disorders
- Post-polio syndrome
- Post traumatic stress disorder (PTSD)
- Postural hypotension
- Reading disorders
- Respiratory disorders
- Schizophrenia
- Spinal cord injuries (levels of injury)
    - Paraplegia
    - Tetraplegia
    - Quadriplegia
- Scar remodeling
    - Hypertrophic scar
    - Wound healing
- Sensory modulation deficits

- Spasticity
- Spina bifida
- Substance use / abuse
- Suicidal ideation
- Tactile defensiveness
- Tardive dyskinesia
- Tendon injury / repair (hand)
- Traumatic brain injury (TBI)
- Tonic bite
- Vision impairments
    - Homonymous hemianopsia
    - Low vision
    - Macular degeneration
    - Retinopathy
- Visual field deficits
- Work-related injuries
- Wound healing (stages)

Intervention Applications / Equipment

- Activities of daily living (ADL)
- Adaptive equipment
- Aging in place
- Allen Cognitive Levels
- Assessment tools (standardized and non-standardized)
- Assistive devices
- Assistive technology (low tech / high tech)
- Augmentative and alternative communication
- Balance training / retraining
- Behavior management strategies
- Biomechanical model
- Body mechanics
- Body scheme awareness
- Cardiac rehabilitation (activities / phases)
- Chaining
    - Forward chaining
    - Backward chaining
- Client-centered approaches
- Cognitive–perceptual intervention strategies
- Community integration
- Community mobility
- Community referrals
- Compensatory techniques
- Coping strategies
- Desensitization techniques
- Developmental play
- Discharge planning
- Durable medical equipment
- Edema management
- Energy conservation
- Endurance exercises
- Environmental adaptation / modification
- Environmental control units (uses / indications)
- Ergonomic principles
- Errorless learning
- Evidence-based practice

- Feeding / swallowing
- Flexibility / stretching exercises
- Functional ambulation
- Goal-setting and prioritization
- Graded activities
- Grasp development / grasp patterns
- Group dynamics / group facilitation
- Handwriting / pre-writing skills
- Home program education
- Injury prevention (educational programming)
- Information gathering strategies
- Interprofessional team collaboration
- Joint protection techniques
- Just-right challenge
- Lifestyle modification
- Memory strategies
- Mobility training
- Motor skills / motor control / motor planning
- Muscle testing
- Observation techniques
- Occupational profile development
- Oral motor skills
- Pain management techniques
- Patient / caregiver education
- Perceptual skill development
- Physical agent modalities (indications / contraindications)
- Positioning (techniques and devices)
- Pressure garments
- Prosthetics (types / functions / uses)
- Purposeful activity
- Range of motion (testing / exercises)
- Reflexes
    - Asymmetrical tonic neck reflex (ATNR)
    - Symmetrical tonic neck reflex (STNR)
    - Labyrinthine
    - Head righting
- Relaxation training
- Risk management (related to service delivery)
- Role playing
- Safety precautions (client and caregiver)
- Seating (types and devices)
- Sensory modulation techniques
- Sensory testing
- Sensory reeducation
- Service competency
- Sequencing skills and abilities
- Social skills
- Splint / orthotic (fabrication / modification)
- Strengthening exercises
- Stress management
- Transfer training / education
- Transition planning
- Trunk control
- Universal design
- Universal precautions

- Visual motor skill development
- Vocational training
- Wellness educational programming
- Wheelchair assessment / modification
- Wheelchair (functional mobility)
- Work hardening / functional capacity
- Work simplification
- Workplace modification

Service Delivery Components (Occupational Therapy Process)

- Activity analysis
- Activity selection
- Assessment (standardized / non-standardized)
- Clinical observation
- Communication skills
- Components of an intervention plan
- Confidentiality
- Conflict of interest
- Conflict resolution

Roles and Responsibilities

- Cultural sensitivity / diversity
- Culturally responsive care
- COTA / OTR roles and responsibilities
- Continuous quality improvement / performance improvement planning
- Discharge planning (processes and procedures)
- Documentation
- Evidence-based practice
- Federally mandated requirements for service delivery
- Frames of reference / models of practice
- Goal-setting / prioritization
- Informed consent
- Insurance authorization / reimbursement
- Intervention planning
- Interviewing skills / methods
- Interprofessional team process
- Listening
- Negotiating
- Outcomes measures
- Professional development activities
- Professional liability
- Program evaluation
- Promoting the profession
- Refusal of service
- Research methods
  - Interpretation of results
  - Reliability
  - Validity
- Research design

- Resource management
  - Time
  - Equipment
  - Supplies
- Risk management
- Screening (standardized / non-standardized)
- Service collaboration
- Service competencies
- Scope of practice
- Strategic planning / goals
- Supervision

Settings/Situations

- Acute care hospital
- Adult daycare center
- Administration / management
- ADA
- Architectural / environmental barriers
- Assisted living facilities
- Automobile / driving
- Bathing / bathroom mobility
- Classroom
- Clinic
- Cooking / meal preparation
- Community-based settings
- Consultant
- Daycare facility
- Dressing
- Early childhood intervention
- Eating / dining
- Grooming / hygiene
- Groups (inpatient / outpatient)
- Group home
- Home health
- Hospice
- IDEA
- Independence
- Inpatient rehabilitation facility
- Interests
- Job site/ vocational / prevocational
- Leisure activities
- Long term care facility
- Occupation
- Playground
- Play activities
- Prison / confinement facility
- School-based
- Skilled nursing facility
- Volunteers
- Wellness programs
- Workplace